KEEP
YOUR
KIDS
THIN

KEEP YOUR KIDS THIN

A Nutritional Handbook for Parents and Children

DR. SEYMOUR ISENBERG

St. Martin's Press   New York

KEEP YOUR KIDS THIN: A NUTRITIONAL HAND-
BOOK FOR PARENTS AND CHILDREN. Copyright
©1982 by Dr. Seymour Isenberg. All
rights reserved. Printed in the United
States of America. No part of this book
may be used or reproduced in any manner
whatsoever without written permission
except in the case of brief quotations
embodied in critical articles or reviews.
For information, address St. Martin's
Press, 175 Fifth Avenue, New York, N.Y.
10010.

Design by Laura Hammond

Library of Congress Cataloging in
Publication Data

Isenberg, Seymour.
  Keep your kids thin.

  1. Obesity in children.   2. Reducing
diets. 3. Children—Nutrition.   I. Title.
RJ399.C6I83   613.2'088054   82-5610
ISBN 0-312-45100-8   AACR2

First Edition

10 9 8 7 6 5 4 3 2 1

2185160

Contents

KING: *Our son shall win.*
QUEEN: *He's fat and scant of breath.*

Hamlet, *Act V, Sc. ii*

KEEP
YOUR
KIDS
THIN

Introduction

IF YOUR BABY COULD TALK

Let's say you are a mother-to-be, settled nicely into your pregnancy, all going well, doing the best you can to have a fine, healthy baby. But are you, really? If your developing child could talk, what would it request of you as a parent? Considering the life-styles and frustrations of millions of children in this country today, chances are your growing embryo would ask you to modify the menu you are dishing up to it. Because—with the best intentions in the world—you may be starting it off on the wrong foot nutritionally. This is something it may be very difficult to make up for later on. You will never again have as much influence over your child as in the so-called "formative years"—and these years begin right in the uterus.

There have been a great many differences of opinion among physicians as to whether the fat baby becomes a fat adult. Lines have been drawn on either side of this argument. My own researches in my Weight Loss Control clinic, talking to thousands of parents, seem to indicate a midway stance in most cases. I do not believe that weight in infancy necessarily indicates later body size. Many overweight—even obese—infants tend to return to a normal weight in childhood; many others, unfortunately, do not. If the parents also are obese, this adds to the possibility of the child or children continuing along this path. Interestingly, however, I have found a more predisposing factor toward a child's obesity to be whether the other children in the

1

family are fat. Even without the parent's overfeeding, a sort of peer pressure appears to exist to make the new child "one of the group."

At the same time, overfeeding is a parental responsibility. The most frequent question I am asked by my patients is, "Doctor, how can I keep my kids from ending up like me?" The answer to that question is the reason why this book has been written. Of course, there is no one answer but rather a multitude of answers, of responses that first you, the parent, and later on the child must make. It is easier for the adolescent or teenager to come to a correct decision about how to eat and what to eat if solid guidelines have been laid down from the beginning.

While I do not believe that the fat baby will of necessity become the fat adult, I do believe that overfeeding in infancy causes a rapid weight gain which, maintained over a long period of time, can lay down the pattern of a future life-style. Your obese son or daughter will give you little thanks for this in the future.

THE MOST FREQUENT MEDICINE—YOURSELF

Control of obesity in children involves a twofold plan. First is to lay down reasonable and easy-to-follow habit patterns while the child is still under parental control. Parental control begins in the uterus and is mostly in the hands of the mother from that point right up through the first two years—though the father is not unimportant here, as I will be pointing out. The second part of the plan is to have a logical followup that the child can pursue on his or her own, one that will be appealing and that will enable the child to resist the peer pressure that is exerted more and more as he or she gradually grows away from the home environment.

You, the parent, have the basic responsibility. Don't kid yourself as far as your kids are concerned. They are awfully smart, no matter how young, so don't try to con them—they can see right through it. How many times have I had an obese mother say to me, "Oh, my son or daughter will never be fat like me. I watch them"? No doubt. But they are also watching you. If it's okay for you to be fat, to eat all that "junk" food, to drink all those sodas—why isn't it okay for them? "Don't do as I do, do as I say," simply doesn't work. It amazes me how many parents still try to get away with that old line. Forget it. In the early stages of life, when basic patterns are being formed, you are the most frequent medicine your child will be taking. You had best be certain it's medicine, not poison, you are furnishing. Strong words? Well, I feel strongly about it. Obesity is running rampant in this country. If the problem is ever going to be brought into focus, it has to be seen right at the grassroots— our young people. To start giving them medicines and maxims as adolescents is not nearly as effective as the dosage of *you* furnished right from the start. Prescribe yourself—and if your image is lacking, do something to change it. Lose weight if you are fat, take up exercise so you will know what it is like when you advise it, change your life-style if it is self-defeating for your children—at least as far as food is concerned. If you are concerned, you can do no less than this. It is just these sorts of changes that are generally overlooked by parents in attempting to deal with their "refractory" children. You shouldn't wait long enough for them to develop difficult habits.

To be effective, any program of therapy dealing with children must involve their peers and their parents. The first steps are in the home—and right at the beginning. Dieting for the parents, even if grossly necessary for their own sakes, is not enough as far as the children are concerned. You must begin to think about changes in your behavior, attitude, and life-style, and if you are afraid that this is too much of a challenge, let me assure you that it isn't really all that difficult. I will be guiding you through certain of these changes in these beginning chapters. All you have to do is to be willing to think about what I have to say and, since it makes sense, follow it. That's the first step. All the other steps will follow easily from there to create an atmosphere in which you, the teacher, will first learn yourself.

That's the point at which, if your developing baby could talk, it might well want to say, "Thank you."

I would like to express my indebtedness to the Institute of Human Nutrition, Columbia University, for much of the scientific research and many of the conclusions regarding food and people in this book.

1
Nutrition: Sense and Nonsense

I'd like to begin with this topic because today it's on everyone's lips. Literally. And much of what you read is either distorted or wrong. Like so many other convoluted subjects, there are not nearly as many "rights" and "wrongs" to nutrition as you might think. Oversimplification seems to be the rule, but this sort of thinking can give you some pretty far-out notions.

First of all, experts on the subject tend to differ among themselves as to what amounts to proper nutrition. Many of these self-styled experts are food faddists who have a particular nutritional supplement to peddle—not for your advantage but for their own. Are these the people who are deserving of your faith? Others are consumer activists busily hopping on the bandwagon of what has become a particularly hot issue; they are more involved with rhetoric than reason. Others are people just looking for a cause; they can be found on almost any side of an argument, giving heated opinions that in the long run amount to just a lot of hot air.

Where does that leave you, the parent, the shopper, who wants to provide the best for your family?

My feeling is that it leaves you with the only person really fit to guide you in nutrition as in any other of your health questions: your family doctor.

YOUR DOCTOR AS NUTRITIONIST

Don't let all the amateur nutritionists sell you a bill of (inedible) goods. While physicians as a group come under criticism for lack of knowledge about nutrition, this is no more than an extension of the idea that a doctor should know everything about everything. It is true that in the past nutrition as such was not taught in medical schools, a fact that is changing rapidly today. But to use this omission as a rallying cry to assert that because of it doctors are the last to express an opinion on the subject is crazy. Of course, not every physician is an expert on the topic. But their qualifications toward expertise are considerably more imposing than those, in most instances, who are making most of the noise. Every physician has had courses in biochemistry, physiology, organic chemistry, and preventive health—to mention just a few subjects that encompass nutritional health. Nutrition is not a new science, despite the efforts that seem to be made to make it appear so. The elements of nutrition—proteins, fats, carbohydrates, vitamins, minerals, and water—have been around a long time. In fact, I know of no course in physiology in which the functions of the body in regard to these elements are not discussed.

So, you see, the principles of nutrition are taught, and always have been taught, in medical schools. They are simply parts of other courses. What is not taught is food composition, how to put all these nutrients together into a palatable and healthy package. A lot of this, of course, is common sense and can be a joint creation between you and your physician—providing he takes the time. This is where many physicians fall down on the job, when they talk about chemicals and nutrients, rather than food, which is what you, the patient, want to talk about. After all, how large is a four-ounce piece of fish, fowl, or meat? How can food be made more appealing even though it is served in smaller portions? What can be done in cooking to make food more appetizing while at the same time have it fill you up more? How can you apply certain principles of behavior modification to foods to help you change your eating habits? How many calories are provided by specific foods, and should you take the calories from these foods or other choices? What about substituting certain foods for others? What about fiber, folic acid, potassium? What about zinc?

All these are questions your family physician is qualified to answer—and, most important, to answer for you and your children's particular needs. You and your children are all individuals and are entitled to be treated as persons, not statistics. Even so, much of what I say can only apply to you, the reader, in a general sort of way. Any questions about anything I say in these pages should be referred by you to your family physician. In the long run, he is always the best one to consult about you, the individual. Should you care to write me, care of the publisher, I will be happy to furnish you with additional information, or clarify a point, to whatever extent I can. I have always done this in my preceeding books and enjoy a lively correspondence with my readers throughout the world.

Having said so much about nutrition in general, let us look at a few specifics. Following are some questions I am frequently asked about food and its effects on the body.

A NUTRITIONAL PRIMER

What is the best food, nutritionwise?

There is really no single food that provides all the nutrients. The body—especially a child's body—works best on a variety of foods. The body, you see, likes to do its own marketing. It shops for its needs among the basic four food groups: (1) meat, poultry, fish; (2) eggs, milk, cheese; (3) fruits and vegetables; (4) grain and fiber foods. Any plan for the growing body should utilize these food groupings for proper nutrition, though amounts can be varied.

How important is portion size?

Nutritionally the amount of a particular food should be adjusted to the individual's needs, not wants. This is standard in any weight loss plan where the portion size has to be calculated to the amount of calories the person is expending. Children do expend lots of calories in their daily activities, though not nearly so much as you might imagine, with TV taking up more and more of their time. My feeling about portion size is that it should be small—divided into two or three ounces—with seconds or thirds possible only after the initial portion has been eaten. I will be discussing this technique further along in the book.

What about alcohol?

On any adult diet there is simply no room for alcohol. As far as children are concerned, the teenage drinker, even one who takes a "moderate" drink, is taking in extra, unneeded calories and, in addition, is increasing his appetite for food. Many teenagers "stick to" beer. This beverage is extremely caloric and should not be used as an alternative to "hard" liquor, at least from a dieting standpoint.

Is it important to have three meals a day?

Not from where I sit. I will be going into this, also, more fully in the course of the book. Many people, children as well as adults, feel bound to the three-meal-a-day regimen whether they are hungry or not. They will also eat "between" meals when hunger strikes. I am going to try to change this habit pattern, make it more convenient to eat, and cut down unnecessary calories accumulated through what I call "clock-watching obesity." I do not believe that breakfast is the most important meal of the day. Believe it or not, the meal that many people are *not* hungry for is breakfast. They eat it because they are afraid to go without it. Adults are afraid they will not have enough energy to get through till lunchtime, and children are afraid they will be yelled at by parents if they don't eat breakfast. During the week they rush through the meal, preferring to spend the extra time in bed. If children really wanted breakfast, all the commercial incentives to eating the meal, such as noisy cereals, colored cereals, and the like, would not exist. Nor would you need all the sweetened breakfast food that abounds in our culture.

Are all calories alike or are there different calories from different foods?

All calories are alike in the laboratory, but they are not alike in the body. The liver does tend to treat certain calories differently than it does others. We will be taking advantage of this fact as we progress into the book. For instance, it has been shown that calories from carbohydrate foods—crackers, sugar—are stored as fat more readily than calories that come from protein such as meat, fish, or fowl. That is not to say that one should then eat these foods exclusively.

What are "empty" calories?

Of course, a calorie is neither "full" nor "empty," since a calorie is really the measurement of a unit of heat. It takes 3,500 calories to make a pound of fat. The expression "full" or "empty" refers to the source from which the calories come. Five hundred calories of ice cream, for instance, are a source more for storage in the body as fat (fuel) than for nutrition as 500 calories of beef, say, would be. The ice-cream calories would then be referred to as "empty" calories, since they are empty of nutritive value—no vitamins, minerals, protein, or fiber being offered to the body.

What about taking extra vitamins and minerals? Do I need them? Do my children need them?

If you are overweight and are going on a plan to lose weight, you probably should take a multivitamin tablet daily. Some of the foods that would not be on your diet plan will be made up for, nutritionally, in this fashion. As far as children are concerned, I do have my patients on a daily vitamin supplement. Despite what many people believe, vitamins do not cause increased hunger.

Since salt is not a food, do I or my children have to stop using it? And isn't salt necessary for life?

Yes, to both questions. This may sound paradoxical but, while salt is necessary to life, you will be getting enough of it in the foods you will be eating to avoid any sodium depletion of your body. On the other hand, overuse of salt via the salt shaker will lead to all sorts of problems, such as water (fluid) retention, hypertension, and salt addiction. There are as many salt as sugar addicts, and addiction to salt is as poor both nutritionally and dietwise as is addiction to sugar. If you are the cook for your family, you should use very little salt. Let the foods be served in as natural a manner as possible. Your family can then salt or not salt according to taste (and salt substitutes are permitted while dieting). If the taste is for oversalting, this must be changed. It is far easier to change this habit in childhood than as an adult; better still, not to let it get started. Incidentally, any salt that is used in a diet should be iodized.

What about zinc and fluorides and these other mini-minerals we keep hearing about?

These elements have little to do with losing weight, though in the case of fluorine, at least, it is essential in the prevention of tooth decay. I am going to be asking all of you—adults and kids—to drink quite a bit of water each day. Fluoridated water is absolutely safe. Just because you are drinking it in greater amounts than usual, don't start believing you are in for trouble. Fluoridated water is perfectly safe for anyone of any age in any state of health. Zinc is another matter. It is a trace element in many foods. I have had no problems with this element in any dietary form I have ever created. However, this does not apply to individuals who are being treated for low zinc. If you are such an individual, you should check with your doctor before going on any sort of diet.

One hears a lot about cholesterol. What is it, exactly, and can children have trouble with high cholesterol as well as adults?

There is a lot of debate as to whether an increase in cholesterol can cause heart attacks. Before going on any diet, or before having any adolescent go on a diet, cholesterol levels should be checked. How to tell if your level is suspect? If you are overweight and eat a lot of eggs and cheese, you could have a cholesterol elevated above the norm. That doesn't mean you have to take drugs to get it down. I have found in my practice that cholesterol levels drop at least 25 percent in the first month as individuals lose weight and change their eating habits. One such eating change involves switching from saturated to unsaturated fatty products. Remember that the cholesterol level (as are many other blood chemistry values) is a range, not a single number. It's a good idea to keep it on the low side of the range.

A NONNUTRITIONAL PRIMER

Old wives' tales abound where nutrition is concerned. Here are some of my favorites, along with my responses to them:

The term "health foods" in supermarket, specialty stores, or what have you means that you have stumbled on a life-giving oasis for special items that will at once reduce you, help you live forever, and will get rid of whatever ailments now afflict you.

In fact, though many of these foods are promoted as having been produced under special conditions—without pesticides and with natural rather than with chemical fertilizers—there's no improvement. I realize I am bringing down on my head the lightnings and thunderings of many of my friends. Yet the truth must be told—and the truth is that plants absorb certain inorganic nutrients (read "chemicals") and that they don't care what the source is, natural or chemical; there is no difference as far as the plant is concerned. The only difference is in your mind—just as St. Joseph and Bayer aspirin are the same compound, the sole difference being in the name. As for the lack of pesticides, studies have shown that even "health foods" contain pesticide traces. In short, all foods are health foods when properly used—and all foods can do you ill when used improperly, no matter how they are prepared or grown.

Processed foods are inferior to the more natural, home-grown variety, since in their manufacture processed foods are somehow diluted of their power.

In general, there is little difference from one to the other, nutritionally. There may be quite a difference in convenience. Processed foods save a great deal of time and work for the homemaker. Heaven knows the person responsible for running the home has enough to do without having to run a mini-farm, starting from scratch with "natural" foods. Don't get too concerned with this particular canard. Processed foods taste so good, with such minimal preparation, that they will never go out of style. Rightly, many proponents of natural foods hold that processed foods make it harder to lose weight because they are so conveniently at hand, and therefore a constant temptation. To this I respond by saying that if you want to lose weight, you can't do it by locking yourself away from food. This was tried with the liquid protein diets of several years ago. Sooner or later you must face the music of those turning lids, popping corks, splashing bottled goods. Without the proper mental attitude, you will never be able to stand it. This is, of course, just as true for kids as adults. It is what goes on in your head as well as what goes into your mouth that counts.

Refined sugar is the snake in the nutritional Garden of Eden. It is poisonous, debilitating, more insidious even than heroin. Why not do away with it?

Because nobody wants to. In fact, nobody has to. Sugar is not all bad. It can be a friend rather than an enemy. It is the abuse of sugar, not sugar itself, that is at fault. It's just easier to blame sugar than oneself.

Research done in recent years at the Monell Chemical Senses Institute at the University of Pennsylania, Philadelphia, has shown clearly that infants are born with a desire for sweets. In fact, even the human fetus exhibits a desire for sweet-tasting fluids. Little wonder then that as children and adults we end up "cheating" on our diets for sugar—whether in pure form or as starch. We are born with a taste for sweets, it isn't something we develop. In a very real sense, therefore, the matter is out of our hands. In a very practical sense, however, we should keep it out of our hands. Unfortunately, none of us fat people do. Or did.

Yet all of us could exist with sugar if we didn't keep making return trips because the stuff tastes so good. Patients tell me, and I know from my own experience, that sugar is addicting. A little bit makes you want more. The problem is, of course, that as a nutrient sugar is completely utilized by the body as a fuel; what can't be burned is stored—as fat. And because of its inborn hold on us, as well as its addictive qualities, and because items made from it tend to be inexpensive, sugar in any number of its forms is the classic fat producer in children. This despite the fact that sugar makes up only 12 to 15 percent of the total calories consumed by adults and only 20 to 25 percent of the total calories consumed by children. A little bit goes a long way. Like alcohol, sugar is not for those who cannot control their craving. For those who can, it is a comfort and a delight. For the makers of the over sixty-two sugar-coated cereals on the market, it is obviously a source of profit. These are your children's enemies—not the sugar. Keep the kids off the breakfast cereals with all their decorative sugar and you will keep them from becoming sugar addicts.

Megavitamin therapy is "in," it seems. And it makes sense, doesn't it? After all, if a little is good, a lot is better.

In fact, are a number of problems better than a few? The irrationality of overdosing oneself or one's children with vitamins is matched only by the statements issued in support of the endeavor. Like any other nutritive element, vitamins should be taken in practical measures, not as some sort of magic.

Speaking of magic, aren't there foods that do special things? Like bananas, prunes, avocados being good for weight loss but bad for cholesterol?

In fact neither bananas nor avocados nor any fruits or vegetables have cholesterol. All of the above-mentioned items are high in potassium, and I use some such foods to supply potassium to my patients on a weight-loss program. Bananas are rather too high in calories to use for a potassium supplement, but cranberries, prunes, and apricots are fine for the job. Avocado is high in vitamin A, and though one contains about 280 calories, half an avocado on a lettuce leaf can be quite a treat to the dieter from the standpoint of variety.

THE BALL IS IN YOUR COURT

If you are a fat parent and you don't want your kids to follow your example, the time has come to really get your head together. It is generally accepted that fat parents have fat children, but it sometimes takes specifics to bring the point home. A recent Public Health Bulletin has reported that on a percentage basis one fat parent will tend to have a 40 percent chance of raising a fat child; with two fat parents, the percentages double. The probability of fat children being raised by normal-weight parents, on the other hand, is only 7 percent. If you are a fat parent, you had better take steps to immunize your children from following your example. The following will help—even if it hurts a bit at first:

1. If it isn't around you can't eat it. Since you may be the one doing the shopping, don't buy foods that you know are taboo. (If you have any question about this, check the lists of regulation foods elsewhere in this book.) If you don't supply it and your children are too young to get it elsewhere, they won't be able to eat it either.

2. Take a few minutes to ask yourself: What did I eat today? How many times did I eat something I wasn't really hungry for?

3. Having considered what you did today, you might try writing down a plan you hope to be able to stick to tomorrow. Writing things down, though it may seem childish, is very helpful. The more important you make the procedure to yourself, the more important it will also be to your kids.

4. TV time is also important. Watching TV during the day with preschool children watching you develops the TV habit in them. Not only does this lead to a sedentary, calorie-storing pattern, but many of the TV commercials glorify junk foods. This is more than enough to establish the desire in children's minds—as the people who write the commercials know well enough. It may seem self-denying, but the less daytime TV the better.

5. Try not to overuse salt at the table and, if you are the cook for the family, don't use too much salt in the cooking process. Needless to say, sugar should not be used at all. As far as sugar substitutes are concerned, if you can do without them, chances are your kids will learn to do without them as

well. If you employ them on a regular basis, my feeling is that you are keeping the desire for sugar only a sword's point away. If you can't do without these substitutes, try using them when the kids aren't watching.

6. Watch out for those midnight snacks. You may think you're sneaking them without anyone seeing you or knowing, but you'd be surprised. Children have ears as well as eyes—and, if it's all right for you to do it, it's equally all right for the kids to follow your example. Remember, they're watching you just as much, and probably more intently, than you are watching them.

7. Do you really need all those second helpings? Why not start a trend in your family—the less the better. As your children grow up, let them get used to the idea that a portion is a finality. They really don't need "more." One assumes that the portion you are dishing out is a healthy one. Keep it that way.

8. The sooner the better. If you are parents of normal weight, you have a head start in the nutrition race. You have the statistics in your favor not to raise a fat child. That doesn't mean you can't raise a fat child. The first child often spells the difference in your life-style. You may begin changing your food habits with this very event. You may stay home more, thereby becoming less active. This can lead to more snacking. This is easy enough to stop once you realize the pattern that is beginning. If you are one of a pair of fat/thin parents, you have a special sort of problem. You may already furnish a poor body image to your child. And, if you are both fat parents, you have practically cooked your child's goose as well as his fate, as I have already pointed out. That is, unless you change your own eating habits—not later on, but now.

If you want your children to be thin and healthy, you will have to be that way yourself. This is true in most cases. That is not to say that thin parents cannot have a fat child. But percentages are against it. Why not tip the scale in favor of your child?

2
Creative
Pregnancy

Time was when a mother-to-be had the notion that pleasant thoughts maintained throughout her pregnancy would lead to a baby that, imbued with these notions, would carry them as an influence through life. On the other end of the spectrum, we have all heard old wives' tales about mothers who were frightened during pregnancy and blamed this for any ill effects on their child. What is more to the point here than maintaining mental equilibrium is physical equilibrium during and even before pregnancy. The effect on your child-to-be can be really dramatic. Here are a few things you as a prospective mother can begin thinking about, both before and during your pregnancy.

A FEW CREATIVE CONCEPTS

Fat is not fair. Fat is not fair to you as a prospective mother, to your baby, or to your obstetrician. Before you even become pregnant you want to be in as good a shape as possible both physically and mentally. If you are merely overweight, lose those few pounds before trying to get pregnant. If you are obese, getting as close as you can to normal weight is essential. It is especially so because obstericians today are not all that pleased about pregnant women "dieting." Once you get pregnant, therefore, you are pretty well stuck with your fat—plus the additional weight you will be gaining throughout your pregnancy. I have had many patients come to me to lose weight

16

after delivery, telling me their obstetricians made no mention to them of the poundage they were putting on. I must emphasize that no pregnant woman should go on a diet without the consent and full knowledge of the physician attending her pregnancy. So, if you think it was unfair of fate to have made you fat before pregnancy, you will find it a lot unfairer—and a lot more uncomfortable—to be fat throughout your pregnancy.

Fat is progressive. As previously mentioned, if you are fat, your children as they grow up may well model their appearances on yours. But it doesn't end there. It is likely that your overweight will go on to haunt the children even after they have begun to leave the home environment and go among their peers. This leads to personality problems, which in turn can lead to further eating as a solace. Let's face it—overweight (let alone obesity) is out of fashion. If you want to be attractive, you've got to be thin, at least reasonably so. About 10 percent of teenagers—girls more than boys—are overweight by whatever method you measure it. Talk about "body image" anxiety. All of this gets worse, of couse, toward the summer, when the bathing suits start coming out of the drawers.

Think thin. While pregnant women are advised to eat a high-quality diet with sufficient calories to allow an adequate physiologic weight gain, this doesn't give you a license to stuff yourself with your favorite goodies in some "medically approved" food orgy. Recently a woman I shall call Mrs. X came to me for weight loss following her delivery. Having gotten her comparatively thin before she became pregnant, I was curious to know how she had managed to put on the eighty-five pounds she now had to lose. "Oh," said she, "my doctor said I shouldn't stint myself. So I went back to eating all those good things you'd taken away from me. I figured it was all right to eat them at that time; I'd make up for it after the baby was born." Well, the baby was born, and now Mrs. X found, to her dismay, that she couldn't deliver the weight she'd gained quite as readily as she'd given birth. "I don't understand," she kept telling me, "I did it the last time much easier." Somehow it is always much easier the last time. That's why the last time should be the last time.

There are definite health hazards in obesity in pregnancy. If you weigh more than 175 pounds in the prepregnant state, you are considered obese. As you get older, and as you continue to become pregnant without losing weight between pregnancies, health risk increases. There are a number of hard facts as far as your physiology goes that produce these statistics. First is the incidence of pulmonary embolism—throwing a clot from poor veins (probably in the legs) into the lungs. The circulatory changes in pregnancy make this possibility all too probable. Next is the incidence of hemorrhage, which rates a close second to pulmonary embolism as the leading cause of death in pregnancy. Not only does the obese woman bleed more readily than the nonobese (because she has more fat, which is an extremely vascular tissue), but the fat itself makes diagnosis and surgical treatment more difficult. Next is the possibility of heart disease. Remember, delivery is a strain on the mother's body. If the heart is already under strain from increased pumping of blood into the excess fatty tissue, additional strain can be too much for it. Last, but not least, is toxemia of pregnancy, more readily haunting the fat than the normal-weight mother.

The above conclusions are based on a review in the *Journal of Obstetrics and Gynecology* of the causes of death in 132 pregnant women. Eighty-four deaths were obstetrically related. Prepregnant weight was greater than 175 pounds in 18 percent of the women, and 12 percent weighed more than 200 pounds. This does not mean that if you weigh 174 pounds you are out of the woods. Not does it mean that if you are overweight you will automatically have a problem delivering. It does indicate that the heavier you are when you get pregnant, the more risk you run. Why bother to run any risk when the solution to the problem is right there in your own hands? And, remember, the time to do it is before you become pregnant.

If you aren't fat when you become pregnant, don't let it happen then. Obviously you are going to gain weight during pregnancy. How much and how fast? A lot depends on you as an individual. You may never have put weight on in your nonpregnant state, so your new metabolism may come as a surprise to you. And don't fool yourself into thinking the weight you gain has to come from your baby and afterbirth. That accounts for only a comparatively small percentage of the total. In general, whether you are of normal weight or obese, a weight gain of over thirty-two pounds is going to be dangerous to your health. One thing to keep in mind is that you can't necessarily go by the height/weight standard that is generally in use. This will not distinguish obesity from overweight resulting from a large or muscular physique. Check with your doctor to determine just what your proper weight is. And once you become pregnant, remember that the developing baby that is now a part of your body is extremely vulnerable to your dietary deficiencies and excesses. One way you can make your baby less vulnerable to them is to become less committed to them yourself.

The trick is not to go to excess either way. In a study that was done by the National Institute of Health, following the course of over 50,000 pregnancies in the United States, it was found that minimum infant mortality rates corresponded with a weight gain of thirty pounds for thin women (that is, women who weighed less than 90 percent of their desirable weight), twenty pounds for normally proportioned women (90 to 135 percent of desirable weight), and sixteen pounds for overweight women. Of all groups, very thin women had the highest infant mortality rates with a low maternal weight gain and the lowest rates with an optimal gain. Interestingly enough, mortality rates varied least with weight gain in obese women, but this group had higher infant mortality rates for most weight gains than the other two groups. Weight gain in the mother seemed to affect male children more than female. Again, what all this means to you is to establish yourself at a reasonable weight before you get pregnant and stay within the range your obstetrician gives you—and make sure he does, indeed, give you such a range. There is no room for ambiguity once you have started on the road to actually having your child.

Don't spoil things once the child is born. Though fat parents tend to have fat children, this does not mean that the trait is inherited, since the same sort of correlation holds true for adopted children and for pets. So, after taking care before and during your pregnancy not to harm your child nutritionally by either under- or overdosing yourself with food, don't forget to hold the good thought after your child is born. It is unfortunately too often the case that children of obese parents grow fatter and fatter until, according to one researcher, by the time they reach age seventeen they generally are three times as fat as those of lean parents.

WHAT ABOUT FAT CELLS?

It seems that individuals who are obese as infants and continue being fat through adolescence probably have more fat cells than people who get fat as adults. In obese children, the fat cells increase continuously from birth to about age fifteen; in lean children, they increase in a sort of spurt—from birth to two years old, then lie dormant till about age ten, then from ten to sixteen they again are formed. Some adults end up with large fat cells, though not a large number; others have many small ones; others have a combination of the two. All of these people are overweight to obese. A lot of the fat-cell situation seems to be guided at the time the baby is being developed in the mother's womb. The children whose mothers have gone on diets within the last three months of their pregnancy, and who are then themselves placed on a restricted diet for the first several months of their life, generally do not have problems with overweight later on. Very possibly this regimen leads to an inhibition of fat-cell development—or, to put it another way, less storage space within the body for fat. Mothers who go on a caloric restriction program early on in their pregnancy—within the first two months, let us say—have children who tend toward overweight and obesity later on.

So you can see how potent the mother's guidance is right from the time of conception. Probably the best idea would be to restrict calories for yourself during the late stages of pregnancy, guided by your obsetetrician. Of course, this doesn't give you the license to overeat during the early stages.

At the same time, don't let all this talk of the fat cells make you think that everything is preordained. It isn't. But your child will need all the help he can get through life in all endeavors, so why not with his fat cells as well? If you, the mother, do not overindulge, your child will have a better chance not to. That doesn't mean that if he ends up with more or larger fat cells than the ordinary he *must* be fat. In obesity control, nothing *must* be. As I have pointed out to many patients, just because you think you have an excess number of fat cells, that's no excuse to fill them with fat. You can have empty closets in your home as well as full ones. A space is only a potential storage. It isn't hard to keep it that way. We will be coming back, in succeeding chapters, to further thoughts on this matter of the fat cells.

LET'S GET SPECIFIC

There's no question that you, the pregnant woman, must have more food in order to meet the demands of your pregnancy so you may have a healthy, normal baby. But, also in order to have a healthy, normal baby, how much and what kinds of food do you eat so that neither you nor your baby will end up fat?

To gain approximately twenty-five pounds during your pregnancy, you would have to increase your caloric intake by about 300 to 500 calories a day. But not just any calories. Not pizza, cake, and ice cream, for instance. These are examples of the "empty calories" I have been at pains to define previously. What you and your developing baby need are nutrients—specifically those from protein, which help build fetal tissues as well as keeping your own in repair. You also need calcium for the development of your baby's bones; iron for making hemoglobin (to help build healthy blood); and folic acid and pyridoxine, two of the B vitamins particularly important to your baby's health. Below is a quick guide for daily food selections that you, the pregnant woman, may use to advantage. My advice is to eat these substances throughout the day rather than limiting them to "three square meals." I have provided a rough estimate as to how the items may be divided up. Remember, it doesn't really matter what your particular food preferences are. We are not talking about your food preferences, a point that must be made absolutely clear. We are talking about food and nutrients. Your so-called favorite foods may well be missing from this guide. Don't even bother to look for them.

A Guide for the Pregnant Gourmet

Necessary Nutrients	Food Involved	Divided through the Day
Protein and iron	Meat, fish, poultry, eggs, legumes/grains, nuts	Try to eat these items 4 or 5 times through the day, in small amounts
Calcium and protein	All forms of milk (skim milk is fine), cheese (not salty), and yogurt	3–4 times a day
Vitamins A and C (including fiber)	Citrus fruits in particular, all fruits to some extent; leafy, red/orange, and green vegetables	Up to 6 times a day in small portions
B vitamins, iron (including fiber)	Whole-wheat products, enriched grain	3 times a day
Water	I advise 8 glasses of water a day (check with your doctor)	1 glass 8 times during a 12-hour period

Eating small "meals" throughout the day will not only give you the basic nutrients your system and baby need, but will avoid your getting uncomfortably full—a situation that can lead to nausea and further eating of starches to alleviate the discomfort. Here, again, is where you may well be taking in excess and "empty" calories.

Two items should be mentioned at this point. The first is the craving for certain foods that can arise during pregnancy. Pickles and ice cream is the classic combination. Such cravings are real enough, but it has been my experience that it is best not to make too much of them. The desire for these strange foods almost always fades once the food is provided, a few bites generally sufficing. But it might be best to allow yourself this much or the desire may continue to haunt you. I have known only a few women who continued to have their craving for odd foods for any substantial length of time. Of course, if you do eat pickles, let us say, throughout your pregnancy, the result could be an alarming fluid-retention. I certainly don't advise giving in to your craving to that extent.

One very unusual type of craving that can occur during pregnancy is called "pica." Here the woman gets an unaccountable desire for such items as chalk, ashes, clay, or earth, even laundry starch—a situation that could prove quite dangerous. If anything like this happens to you, see your doctor immediately so he can check into it. At least two women have told me they had developed such symptoms during their pregnancy but assumed that it was because there was some nutrient lacking in their "regular" diet. Fortunately, no harm came from it in either case. However, there are no nutrients in earth or clay or chalk that your body requires, and the craving for such nonfoods during pregnancy is still something of a medical mystery.

The second of the two items I mentioned is far more common than the craving for exotic or nonfoods. This problem is exemplified by the obese woman who says to me, "Doctor, I was never heavy until I got pregnant. It started with my first baby and with each additional pregnancy I got fatter. So, you see, it isn't really my fault."

Well, if we get right down to it, obesity does not come about because of anybody's fault. I do not subscribe to the opinions that categorize obesity as an affliction of weak-willed or "inferior" individuals. In my years of treating obese individuals, I have noted among them the same gradations of intellect as in the nonobese population. People really do not, in the main, become obese because they go out of their way to make pigs of themselves. In fact, the average complaint of most obese people is "Doctor, I don't eat that much."

As for the obese woman who blames her pregnancy for her condition, there is a possibility that she could be right. I'm not talking now of the mothers who eat everything in the book during their pregnancy and claim they "watch themselves." They are, indeed, watching themselves. They are watching themselves eat. No, I'm talking about the nonobese woman who gets pregnant, gains a normal amount of pregnancy weight, and following delivery cannot lose it. Research has lately begun to show there may be a specific physiological reason for this. See chapter 4 for more information on this.

NUTRIENTS FOR YOUR BABY

The pregnant woman is eating for two, and it therefore behooves you to choose your foods even more carefully than you would just for yourself. Your basic *calories* should come from meat, fish, poultry, fats, fruits, grains, and legumes. Nuts can be eaten in moderation, provided they are not salty. In fact, salt should be used with moderation. Follow your doctor's advice in this as well as in the number of calories you take in. I emphasized the word "calories" above because overweight people tend to look askance at the word, as though there were something old-fashioned about it, as though (as one book stated in its title years ago) calories don't count. There's nothing old-fashioned about watching your calories. And they certainly do count. They'll count you out if you aren't careful. Choose your caloric ration from among the foods enumerated, but I suggest you eat them in small amounts throughout the day rather than limiting them to mealtimes. This is a good habit to get into before you become pregnant and to continue thereafter. It is one of the most potent weapons in the arsenal of the overweight. Eat slowly, chew well, and take your calories in small portions as your body tells you it wants them, not as society has dictated you must divide them. Think: Am I hungry? If the answer is yes, then eat until you are comfortable. Don't stuff yourself until you are "full." You aren't a gas tank in a car, after all.

To the foods enumerated above you may add eggs, milk, and milk products—although I suggest you don't overdo these items. Both these substances and the ones listed above are a source of protein. You need a substantial amount of protein when you are pregnant, since this material is the actual fabric of your baby's body and lack of it will cause difficulties with its normal development. Keep in mind that not only is your baby being formed, but the afterbirth is as well. Many mothers tend to think of the afterbirth, or placenta, as something that comes along when the baby is ready to be born. It is formed together with the developing embryo, and lack of sustenance for this crucial pipeline to the mother's body can have a weakening effect on the embryo. Women who go on "crash" or "fad" diets early on in pregnancy—that is, within the first three months— can cause problems to the placenta.

Calcium is probably the most important element for the pregnant woman. Many doctors furnish it in pill form. It's more fun—and, from the standpoint of learning to live with food, more fulfilling—to take it in the form of food. About 1,200 mg a day is recommended, and you can acquire it in yogurt, cheese (nonsalty—I like cottage cheese), and leafy green vegetables. I emphasize these items; most people think of milk as a source of calcium, which it is, but I would like you to chew rather than drink. While you can supplement your calcium requirements with milk, it would be nice to deemphasize this source, which will not satisfy hunger nearly as well as something you can literally get your teeth into.

Next to calcium, the elements most necessary are iron, folic acid, and pyridoxine (vitamin B_6). Liver, foods cooked in an iron pan, leafy green vegetables, whole grains, wheat germ, meats, fish, and poultry are good sources. I have purposely left out of my table (see page 22), for all the items enumerated, many foods that also contain them but that add calories you may not need. Rather than go ahead and eat these foods, ask your doctor to supplement the requirements I have listed. You certainly don't want to have to live on pills; as I have said, it is far more satisfactory all the way around to get as many as possible of your nutrients from food. But pills do furnish nutrients without calories, and according to your weight as well as your needs, you may want to utilize supplementation. In fact, you may have to. Iron, for instance, is present in marginal amounts in many diets, and the obese or overweight woman may be deficient in this substance even before pregnancy begins. Calcium, though present in large amounts in many foods, including "diet" foods, may not be taken into the body chemically if large amounts of phosphorus are also present—which is often the case in processed foods. Folic acid is, on the other hand, very scarce in the general run of foods most people eat. For women who were taking contraceptive pills, body reserves of both folic acid and vitamin B_6 are probably already low.

So all those prenatal supplements are necessary. Many women have said to me, "I'm afraid to take those pills. Won't they give me an appetite?" when referring to prenatal supplements. This is one of those old wives' tales that simply isn't so. Yet it is always disconcerting to me to observe how many of my patients, once they become pregnant, use these prenatal supplements as an excuse to eat. "They make me so hungry," one lady confessed to me just the other day. But is it really hunger? Stop and think. There's an important pill that will help you do your thinking if you'll use it. It sits on top of your neck. The sensation you feel may not be hunger. It may be greed. It is important for you to learn to distinguish between the two. We will be discussing the difference between them as we go along.

A FEW QUESTIONS YOU MAY WANT TO ASK

I've chosen some of the questions I have found come up most often and have tried to answer them as succinctly as possible.

What do I do when I feel sick to my stomach and the only thing that will relieve it is something like crackers or bread? I almost always get sick in the first month or so.

It is difficult to enumerate any substitutions for things that settle a particular stomach, since what works well for one woman may not work for another. I have to assume, therefore, that you have tried everything else and cannot substitute the above items. But you can, at least, try to make them as little caloric as possible, since you are taking them "medicinally," if I may so express it. Choose crackers that are low in calories—you can easily check these in any listing. You might even try dietetic crackers; certainly you can use saltless ones. As for bread, I have found that the more chewable, the better. The crust from Jewish rye works very well in this regard. Don't work your way through the bread to the crust, as one woman did. Cut the crust off and chew on it slowly. And, most important, once the nausea goes stop eating. It isn't necessary to finish the box of crackers or the loaf of bread just because you've gotten started on it—any more than you would drink the whole bottle of cough syrup. Just take your "dose."

Should I take water with my meals or in between? And won't I swell up with too much water?

I try to get away from the idea of eating meals. I feel you should eat throughout the day when you are hungry—small amounts of the foods enumerated rather than fairly large amounts at designated intervals. Water can be taken at any time: with meals, as well as between them. As far as swelling from water is concerned, the edema of pregnancy comes about from causes other than water drinking. Any sort of swelling is a situation your doctor should check; if he feels you are taking in too much water, he will tell you. Healthy kidneys work best on water, not diet soda, regular soft drinks, alcohol, or juice. Your body tends to lose water more through the skin than the urinary bladder. In my opinion, the most neglected item on the pregnant woman's list is water. As I state in the table on page 22, I feel that eight 8-ounce glasses a day is not too much; again, your own doctor should be your guide.

I am overweight by about twenty-five pounds. I've been on a very good diet—in fact, I've lost five pounds in the last week. I find now that I'm pregnant. Is it safe for me to continue on a diet?

I feel it is probably best for you to see your obstetrician and follow whatever diet he may prescribe. The fact is, pregnancy is quite enough for any woman to handle by itself, without the possible complication of trying to lose weight as well. Wait until the baby is born and then breastfeed; this should help you to quickly return to your prepregnancy weight. If this is still too heavy a weight for you, you may then return to a diet specifically for weight loss.

I am a pregnant teenager. I have always had a weight problem and now, with the baby, I'm afraid I'm really going to blow up. What should I do to avoid this?

Both you and your baby are growing. Your nutritional needs, to say nothing of your baby's, require an adequate amount of nutrients to keep you both in good health. You should be taking in about 2,400 calories a day, most of it proteins. However, you should be guided in this by your obstetrician. A varied diet, still emphasizing protein, will keep you from becoming bored yet will still emphasize the necessity of taking in those vital nutrients. Again, after delivery, you should take immediate steps to lose whatever weight you have gained through your pregnancy—and make sure you don't become pregnant again until you have lost it.

I am a vegetarian. I am also fat. I am also pregnant. My friends seem amazed to find that a vegetarian can get fat. Is this really so unusual? And what will happen to the baby if I want to remain a vegetarian throughout my pregnancy?

Your first question first. No, it is not unusual for a vegetarian to become obese, though the mystique involved in being a vegetarian seems to make it hard for nonvegetarians to believe. I have treated many overweight people who have been vegetarians for a long time before ever coming to me. As for your second question, it should not hurt your baby in the least for you to remain on a vegetarian regimen. Your doctor may advise you to increase your intake of such foods as legumes and beans, since these are the major vegetable sources of protein. He will probably take blood tests to check your cholesterol level, especially if eggs are a large part of your routine. You will also probably need supplements such as iron, calcium, folic acid, and vitamins B_6 and B_{12}. These are found only in animal products such as meat, eggs, and milk products, which you may not eat on your particular vegetarian plan.

What I am worried about mostly as a fat pregnant woman is the pregnancy poisoning I hear so much about. To avoid this I've decided to go on a very strict diet during my pregnancy and avoid salt. Will this help?

What you are talking about is the toxemia of pregnancy, which is by no means as common as you seem to believe. When it occurs it produces high blood pressure, retention of fluid—called "edema"—and loss of some plasma proteins from the blood. This loss will show up in the urine, a condition called "proteinuria." Whether or not restricting calories actually prevents toxemia of pregnancy is debatable; some doctors think it aids its occurrence. As far as salt is concerned, my feeling is that you should limit it during your pregnancy, toxemia fear or not, just as a matter of good health. Salt will increase the possibilities of your becoming edematous (retaining water).

I know this isn't a nutrition question, but what about drinking and/or smoking during pregnancy? Will these have an effect on my baby? I'm afraid if I don't smoke I'll put on even more weight.

A lot depends on how heavily you indulge in these two activities. Heavy alcohol consumption will put weight on you and may interfere with your baby's growth pattern to the extent that the baby becomes retarded or suffers other birth defects. Other subtle abnormalities may not turn up for months or even years after birth. Since it is really impossible to postulate a "small" or "reasonable" amount of alcohol that is "safe," I like to play it safe and say "No alcohol during pregnancy." That is the only safe way I have ever found. As for smoking, the same thing holds. Excessive smoking (which I consider as more than half a pack of cigarettes a day) may cause almost as many problems with the developing baby as alcohol. So, you see, your question does involve nutrition.

YOU ARE WHAT YOU EAT—
AND SO IS YOUR BABY

I would like to use the following illustration to show how effectively poor nutrition can sabotage your growing baby. One of the most difficult jobs I have is convincing people that just because they don't feel anything out of the way happening during pregnancy, damage can still be done because of poor nutrition on their, the mother's, part. A recent study in Wales has linked a specific birth defect of the neural tube (the developing spinal cord) to what the mother does or does not eat. In one area 103 women who had already given birth to children with neural tube defects were given an hour and a half of dietary counseling before 109 pregnancies. The women were advised to cut their intake of refined sugar, potato chips, potatoes, cream buns, sweets, and soft drinks and to make sure they had plenty of protein. In another area, 77 women were not given such advice during their 77 pregnancies. The dietary counseling led 78 of the 103 women in the first area to improve their diet; most of the uncounseled women did not. Only 3 babies born to women who had been counseled had neural tube defects—and these 3 women had not changed their diet based on what they had been told. Previously, all of these women had had a child born with the defect. Of the uncounseled women, 5 had a second child born with a neural tube defect.

For any woman who has delivered a baby that has a birth defect of any sort, dietary counseling is recommended. If you get nothing out of this book but that one idea, it will be well worth while. If there is a history in your family of any such pregnancies, again counseling would be a good idea. It is hard to convince people that what they are used to eating, drinking, or smoking may have a deleterious effect on the unborn child, but such is indeed the case. I was almost going to say, "Don't take it personally." But I think you have to take it personally. It's the person inside you who will be getting the brunt of your poor eating habits. Certainly, he or she will take it personally.

SOME SAMPLE PREGNANCY MENUS
FOR THE OVERWEIGHT MOTHER

I feel that how you eat is more important than what you eat—though this doesn't mean what you eat doesn't matter, as the foregoing discussion must clearly show. Remember to have small meals through the day rather than one large one at night. Eat more to satisfy hunger than simply because it is that time of the day. It is true that you are eating for two; that means you must make your food choices twice as carefully, not that you must automatically eat twice as much of all the "wrong" things. When you eat, eat slowly and enjoy it. Try to concentrate on your food rather than on what is going on around you, as this may prove distracting and allow you to fall back into bad habits. Although I divide the menus below into breakfast, lunch, and dinner, I would have you think of these as items that can be eaten any time you are hungry. Don't consider particular items as belonging to a specific time of the day. Eat only when your hunger, not the time of day, demands you eat.

SAMPLE MENU 1

BREAKFAST

4 ounces orange juice
1 serving bran flakes with raw or cooked (canned) peaches (may use cooked without the juice; may use part of milk for cereal)
8 ounces whole milk

LUNCH

4 ounces V-8 or tomato juice
Egg salad on 3 lettuce leaves (mash eggs; use vinegar and oil, pepper to taste, no salt, chop in celery, raw onion)
3 tomato slices
2 pieces Ry-Krisp

DINNER	8 ounces chicken (white meat) or 8 ounces nonoily fish (broiled)
	Carrot/apple salad (1 apple, 1 carrot, raw; chop roughly, mix with lemon juice, 2 teaspoons diet mayonnaise)
	1 small baked potato (no butter, no salt, may eat the skin)
	½ cup cooked broccoli or cauliflower
	Coffee, tea
SPEED SNACKS (optional—choose any two throughout the day)	1 cup plain yogurt, 2 carrot sticks
	2 slices American cheese on 2 pieces Ry-Krisp
	1 raw pear or three prunes

Sample Menu 2

BREAKFAST	½ grapefruit
	1 cup cooked oatmeal
	8 ounces skim milk (may use part for oatmeal)
LUNCH	1 apple, raw or baked
	1 six-ounce-size hamburger on 1 piece whole-wheat bread
	Salad (3 lettuce leaves, 3 slices tomato), with any commerical oil and vinegar dressing
	Coffee, tea
DINNER	6 ounces lamb or veal (baked, broiled, fried in nonstick pan)
	½ cup cooked corn (not creamed)
	4 cooked asparagus stalks
	4 ounces apple juice (unsweetened)

SPEED SNACKS
(optional—choose
any two throughout
the day)

2 tablespoons peanut butter and
diet jelly on 2 pieces Ry-Krisp
1 cup plain yogurt
3 tablespoons low-fat cottage
cheese with 1 whole sliced
orange

SAMPLE MENU 3

BREAKFAST

8 ounces grapefruit juice
⅔ cup cornflakes
8 ounces skim milk (may use part
for cereal)
1 egg, boiled or poached
Coffee, tea

LUNCH

4 ounces roast beef
1 slice whole-wheat bread
Salad (celery, watercress, tomato,
escarole, cucumber) with 1
tablespoon diet French dressing
8 ounces whole milk

DINNER

4 ounces shrimp or 8 ounces
nonoily fish (broiled or fried in
nonstick pan)
1 cup cooked brussels sprouts,
cauliflower, or broccoli
1 small potato, boiled or baked
(no butter)
½ cup plums (canned, without the
juice)
Coffee, tea

SPEED SNACKS
(optional—choose
any two throughout
the day)

1 small banana
½ cup low-fat cottage cheese on
    lettuce leaf
8 ounces tomato or V-8 juice

SAMPLE MENU 4

BREAKFAST

1 orange, sliced
⅔ cup cooked Wheatena
8 ounces skim milk (may use part
    for cereal)
Coffee, tea

LUNCH

1 cup cottage cheese
6 ounces broiled nonoily fish
Tossed salad (sliced tomato, green
    pepper, mushrooms, shredded
    lettuce; 2 cups total) with 2
    tablespoons oil and vinegar
    dressing
½ cup stewed plums
8 ounces whole milk

DINNER

8 ounces roast chicken, turkey, or
    veal
1 cup cooked brussels sprouts,
    broccoli, or spinach
½ cup cooked turnips
½ cup small boiled onions
1 slice regular bread
½ cup unsweetened fruit cocktail

SPEED SNACKS
(optional—choose
any two throughout
the day)

4 prunes

2 tablespoons (total) peanut butter
and diet jelly on 2 pieces Ry-
Krisp

1 raw apple, orange, or pear

SAMPLE MENU 5

BREAKFAST

8 ounces orange juice
1 egg (boiled or poached)
1 small roll
Coffee, tea

LUNCH

1 cup cottage cheese
½ cup grapefruit sections
1 frankfurter or 1 six-ounce
hamburger (either on 1 slice
regular bread)
8 ounces skim milk

DINNER

8 ounces lamb, veal, or turkey
(baked, broiled, fried in
nonstick pan)
1 medium slice cranberry sauce
Tossed salad (shredded lettuce,
cucumber, carrots, 3 slices
tomato; 2 cups total) with 2
tablespoons oil and vinegar
dressing
1 small potato, boiled or baked
(no butter)
½ cup cooked peas or corn (not
creamed)
1 raw apple or pear
Coffee, tea

SPEED SNACKS
   (optional—choose
   any two throughout
   the day)   1 small banana
                                   1 cup unsweetened fruit cocktail
                                   1 cup plain yogurt

SAMPLE MENU 6

BREAKFAST   4 ounces orange juice
                                   ⅔ cup oatmeal
                                   1 egg (boiled or poached)
                                   1 cup skim milk (may use part for
                                      cereal)
                                   1 small roll
                                   Coffee, tea

LUNCH   2 thin slices ham
                                   1 cup cooked spinach
                                   2 pieces Ry-Krisp
                                   ¼ slice cantaloupe or 1 raw apple

DINNER   4 ounces shrimp cocktail
                                   8 ounces sirloin steak (broiled)
                                   ½ cup potato (fried in nonstick
                                      pan)
                                   ½ cup cooked turnips, broccoli, or
                                      cauliflower
                                   Tossed green salad (2 cups total)

SPEED SNACKS
   (optional—choose
   any two throughout
   the day)   4 prunes
                                   1 cup plain yogurt
                                   1 raw apple

SAMPLE MENU 7

BREAKFAST

½ grapefruit
⅔ cup cornflakes
1 egg (boiled, poached, or fried in nonstick pan)
2 pieces Ry-Krisp with 2 tablespoons diet jelly
8 ounces skim milk (may use part for cereal)

LUNCH

1 cup low-fat cottage cheese
1 four-ounce hamburger on 1 slice regular bread with 1 teaspoon ketchup and 1 slice raw onion
3 lettuce leaves
1 cup unsweetened fruit cocktail

DINNER

4 ounces shrimp or crabmeat cocktail
8 ounces flounder or similar nonoily fish
1 small baked potato
½ cup cooked cauliflower, spinach, or broccoli
Tossed green salad (2 cups total) with 2 tablespoons oil and vinegar dressing
Coffee, tea

SPEED SNACKS
(optional—choose any two throughout the day)

1 cup plain yogurt
1 small banana
4 prunes

The above sample menus are just that—samples. They are suggestions only, to be modified, approved, or rearranged by your doctor according to your personal needs. Yet, they are specific.

They will provide you with a point of departure for the foods that you will eat each day. Some obstetricians provide their patients with very general lists. Such diets are so ambiguously confusing—involving all sorts of food groups, substtution lists, special instructions, general instructions, exchange ratios—that many patients find them too bewildering to follow. Here I have given you some concrete examples. It is simple enough for you, with your doctor's help, to take it from there. Let's keep it simple, for heaven's sake!

3
A Vegetarian View

Before your baby is born, your body supplies it with essential nutrients. After your baby is born, if you are breastfeeding, your body is still a major supplier of nutrients. A movement that is becoming more and more popular in Western society at this time is vegetarianism. One of the questions I am asked frequently on interviews and during lectures involves precisely this life-style. I would like to discuss vegetarianism and its effect on both the mother and the baby, predelivery and directly thereafter. If you are not a vegetarian, you may still find this chapter of value in its discussion of vegetarian supplementation of "regular food."

SO YOU'RE A VEGETARIAN

You may already be a vegetarian or are thinking of becoming one. How will this affect you as a pregnant woman or as a nursing mother? First of all, the so-called vegetarian diet, is really not a diet at all but simply an alternation of the "regular" eating patterns. Those who eat foods only from plant origin are called "vegans"; those individuals who add to this dairy products and eggs are called "ovo-lacto vegetarians." If you take only dairy, no eggs, you are a lacto-vegetarian. Let me say immediately that all these vegetarian diets are fine and will provide adequate amounts of all essential nutrients when properly balanced. And don't fool yourself—vegetarians can also get fat.

The chief difficulty with the vegan diet is the necessity to meet the body's protein requirements, since the proteins present in plants are not always sufficient to do this. This is especially true for adolescents. Certain vegetable combinations must be added to the diet to meet the protein needs of the vegan: cereals, beans, and peas in specified amounts. Check with your pediatrician for specific guidelines.

WEANING YOUR CHILD TO VEGETARIANISM

"The family that eats together stays together" may well become a slogan of the future. At least this is so where the diet acts as an emotional bind. For many vegetarians, this is certainly the case. Vegetarianism may become as much a mental discipline as a simple choice of foods based on taste. For the infant, unable to choose for him or herself, however, the primary interest is strictly physical: how well can his or her body thrive, given (1) a nursing mother who is a vegetarian, and (2) that the infant is him or herself a vegetarian.

For the nursing vegetarian mother, very little problem exists as long as she maintains a balanced diet. However, with the increased trend to "vegan," or "complete" vegetarian, families, more and more small children are being weaned to diets of pure plant origin. Such a child is particularly susceptible to protein-calorie malnutrition. That does not mean the child cannot exist as a vegetarian, but that the mother must continue the use of soy-based milk or milk products beyond the weaning period. As for solid food, peanut butter, soybeans, or lentils can be used. The rate of growth of any child in a vegan family must be closely watched to make certain he or she is getting adequate dietary protein. Adequate Vitamin B_{12}, which aids the body in red blood cell production, is another possible problem. Unfortunately, one can go without B_{12} for a long time before symptoms develop; in a child this could lead to an alarming situation even more so than in an adult. The solution is simple—preventive care. Certain breakfast cereals are "fortified" with vitamins, among them B_{12}. Brewer's yeast is also a source. B_{12} can be given by injection—though this is not, certainly, a popular method with the kids—and can also be taken in tablet form, provided a set schedule is followed.

Iron and calcium must also be adequate in the vegan diet of both adults and children. Certain vegetable foods are higher in iron than are others: kidney beans, white rice, and banana are among the best in this regard. During certain periods in life iron supplements are necessary in people who are strict vegetarians. These times include pregnancy, early childhood, and adolescence. In addition, any major loss of blood, including a donation of blood to others, requires that the vegetarian donating be put on iron tablets.

Calcium-high foods include hard cheese, leafy greens, almonds, and—the highest source—milk and yogurt.

SOME VEGETARIAN DIET SUGGESTIONS

As I have said, the main concern with being a vegetarian is getting the right amount of protein. This means both quality and quantity. The Recommended Dietary Allowances (RDA) for protein are:

Daily RDA (in grams)

Infants	0–1	13
Children	1–3	23
	4–6	30
	7–10	34
Males	11–14	45
	15+	56
Females	11–18	46
	19+	44
	Pregnant	30+
	Lactating	20+

It is not at all difficult, using such foods as grains, legumes, milk products, eggs, vegetables, nuts, and seeds, to feed one's family and oneself the correct amount of protein as indicated above without consuming any meat whatsoever. Since almost all vegetables contain approximately 2 grams of protein per ½ cup cooked serving, these foods add to the total available protein per day.

Meals or, rather, "food blocks" made on a basis comparable

to those developed in the preceding chapter would involve many of the same foods without the meat and fish. Peanut butter, pot cheese, and nonfat dry milk are staples, of course, and any food is made tastier with the addition of seasonings, such as cinnamon or other flavorings or herbs, which certainly need not be caloric.

A word about peanut butter. This should be eaten without bread—and any jelly must be diet. Peanut butter in small amounts is quite nutritious; a tablespoon with one or another of the food blocks on a vegetarian menu is not going to sabotage weight loss. If overused, of course, it can add too many calories. It is, all the same, a valuable source of protein.

SNACKING AND ITS ADVANTAGES

I would like to make it clear that I am not against snacking. In fact, I prefer "snacking" to meals. We tend to snack when we are hungry; we tend to eat meals because we feel we have them coming. We tend to look on snacking as "bad" but on meals as "good." We even, in most "diet" plans, follow the course of three meals a day with no between-meals snacking.

I'd like to turn that way of doing things around. I'd like you not to eat meals, but instead to snack. Make sure you are hungry when you snack. Don't eat meals as such. Turn your meals into snacks. This can be as well accomplished on the vegetarian diet as on any other. Snacking is the key to making sure children and adolescents get enough calories but not the surplus that the addition of meals with such snacks would provide. Light protein snacks taken through the day are the key to satisfying hunger. In addition, I suggest (especially with children) that finger foods be used. There is a great deal of relating to food that happens through the sense of touch. There are tricks you can play on your mouth, for instance, that will fool it into thinking it is getting more food than is actually going in. For example—and this is especially effective with children—the wider the mouth opens, the more psychologically filling is the result, the end result being that mouth hunger is more quickly satisfied. Items that tend to make the mouth work more are therefore to be preferred for snacks. "Treats" like celery stuffed with cottage cheese or a small amount of peanut butter serve well in this regard. Finger foods provide a direct relationship with the food and make it seem that more is being taken in.

To give another example, if you were to eat a piece of lettuce and a slice of American or Swiss cheese from a plate, using a fork, you would likely find it far from an exhilarating experience. Certainly you cannot expect a child to sit still for this sort of food engagement. Nor would mouth or stomach be particularly satisfied at the conclusion.

But take that same lettuce leaf and piece of cheese and roll the cheese up in the lettuce. Now you have a "sandwich" for which your mouth must open fairly wide—and you must hold it in your fingers. You'll be surprised to find how satisfactory this sort of sandwich can be—and how challenging making these items can be for the child. Whether vegetarian or "regular" food fancier, there are things you can do with snacks and foods to prevent hunger and also lose weight. For the child who shows a tendency to put weight on, or for one who is already in serious trouble, no excuse about the type of food will serve. Use the foods that are within the range of whatever nutrition plan you favor. Imagination and snacking can turn a potentially dangerous situation into a thoughtful and selective weight-loss plan by employing food as a friend, not an enemy!

4
Feeding Your New Baby

Okay. You've gone through your nine months of pregnancy and the delivery and the hospital and you are determined to lose the weight that you have put on during the pregnancy. But what about your baby? What sort of figure is he or she going to cut? How can you start, right at the outset, to prevent your baby from ever being faced with the weight problem you may have been fighting all your life?

BREAST IS BEST

Many women who have trouble losing pounds gained during pregnancy would be better off breastfeeding after delivery. If they would begin this regimen right after the first pregnancy, they might very well be able to avoid carrying a weight gain from one pregnancy into a succeeding one. Breastfeeding, for many women, seems to help bring the body down to a "normal" weight and statistics are coming in that tend to back this up. Breastfeeding will also give your baby the proper first steps along the road to proper nutrition.

It is important to remember that the fat baby is not the healthy baby. It is almost impossible to convince most grandmothers of this, and for many mothers it is often easier to give in to grandmotherly demands that the child eat, eat, eat than have a continual running battle. But the battle involves your child's health. Breastfeeding will, at least initially, give you the last word in this particular argument. However, there are other reasons as well.

One very good one is that milks of different species are far from being all the same. They are, in fact, highly complex mixtures, each mammal having its own specifics tailored to its own particular needs. Whale milk, for instance, is higher in fat and calories than almost any other milk. Rabbit milk is very high in protein. Young whales, living in cold water, need the high fat and calories; young rabbits need the high protein for a very rapid, early growth.

The differences between the milk of cows and that of humans also reflect some of the basic differences between those two species. Calves tend to double their birth weight in one third the time that human infants do, mostly because cow's milk contains three times more protein than human milk.

Whether the developing baby bred on cow's milk can use all that extra protein is a question of some debate. Not so debatable is the work being done in many laboratories that suggests that human milk is particularly suitable for rapid brain growth. Also, its pattern of certain types of fatty acid parallels that in human brain tissue. Human milk also varies a lot from one woman to another; it is quite possible that an individual woman's milk may be especially suited to her own baby's nutritional needs.

Commercial formulas have been modified in many instances in an attempt to duplicate human milk. To the extent that the basic ingredients are known—protein, mineral content, etc.— this may be mimicked. But there are components in human milk that have not been analyzed enough to duplicated. Then, there's the problem with getting the mix just right. All in all, it's not quite so easy as you may think—or as some of the advertisements for "humanized" cow's milk may have led you to believe. In addition no formula can imitate the anti-infective properties of human milk.

So there are a number of reasons, other than getting a fat baby, that would bring the breast into play. But let's have another look at some statistics regarding the fat baby.

Studies seem to indicate that, on the average, bottle-fed infants are larger and heavier at the age of one year than are breastfed babies. Now you may be one of those holding the opinion that this is all to the good; that here we have a robust, healthy infant developing rapidly and therefore ahead of the game. What is usually forgotten (if, indeed, many people bother to think about it at all) is that such weight gains in bottlefed babies are all too often disproportionate to length gains. In breastfed babies the two measurements tend to be in better balance. What I'm getting around to saying is that bottle-fed babies get fatter than breastfed ones. And, as I keep repeating, childhood obesity seems to have a direct relationship to the overweight infant. Childhood obesity, in fact, seems to point backward to the hefty baby, and forward to the obese adult with all his or her associated medical problems.

But let's look at this just a little closer. Why should the breastfed baby have less chance to become obese than his bottlefed cousin—or brother or sister, for that matter, since I have often run into family situations where, out of four children, all but one was obese—and that thin one had been nursed on the breast. There are good and reasonable explanations for this. For one very important reason, breastfed babies are more in control of the feeding situation than those on the bottle. When they are full, they stop sucking and that's the end of the feeding for that time. Bottlefed infants, on the other hand, are all too often urged to finish the bottle (many mothers insist on calling the bottle the "feeding" and feel insecure unless this feeding has been completed). But your baby may no longer be hungry, and encouraging it to finish its bottle is imparting into it a taste for food above and beyond hunger that it will carry into child- and adulthood. Eating for the sake of eating is what makes us all obese. Like so many of the things we do, this, too, starts in childhood.

Another reason for bottlefed babies becoming obese more often than breastfed babies is that they are usually started on solid foods earlier than the breast nursers. This is a great factor contributing to overweight. Most solid foods are equipped with more calories per gram than either infant formulas or human milk. Nursing infants also have a harder job getting their milk— they have to expend more energy at this than they would have to do from the bottle. Interestingly, it has been noted that breastfed infants spend more time awake and less time in a crib than those who are bottlefed. Although it is hard to make generalizations, one might reasonably conclude that the breast baby was more alert than the bottle baby because of some component of the breast milk, and that the bottle baby's food was more "alien" to it.

And, since obesity is in great part a psychologic entity, it would seem that the breast baby is more secure than the bottlefed one. The mother-infant interaction appears to be more enhanced with a breastfeeding relationship. The breastfeeding woman will tend to touch her baby, rock it, and sleep with it to a far greater extent than the woman who is bottlefeeding. While there is no reason why the bottlefeeding mother cannot do the same thing, it is not quite so much a matter of course as with the breastfeeder.

One point that may or may not be valid is that breastfeeding provides more sensory stimulation to the baby than does bottlefeeding. This allows the infant to get the maximum enjoyment from the food. Such children tend to be slower eaters as they grow up, able to get their oral satiation from smaller amounts of food than their obese peers, who seek in vain the same satisfaction from more.

SOME MYTHS ABOUT BREASTFEEDING

Since there are myths about everything else, why not about breastfeeding too? Here are a few of them you may or may not be familiar with:

Breastfeeding prevents cancer in the mother. There is no evidence that breastfeeding prevents cancer. If that's your reason for doing it, fine. You'll reap other gains—and so will your child. But your basic notion is probably incorrect.

Breastfeeding increases the cancer risk for female babies. There is no evidence that breastfeeding transmits breast cancer or any other type.

Breastfeeding serves as a contraceptive, so it is safe to have intercourse during this time. Well, yes and no. Yes, the breastfeeding woman may not ovulate. But this is an unreliable crutch at best, since individuals vary in suppression of ovulation. It is best to use a more reliable method of birth control than breastfeeding. I know, personally, at least three women who became pregnant during lactation.

Breastfeeding will spoil a woman's figure—particularly sagging breasts. Again, this is dependent more on individual variation than anything else. Pregnancy, not nursing, primarily changes the shape and texture of the breasts. Whether a woman nurses or not, breasts that were quite upright before pregnancy can sag. On the other hand, I have known nursing mothers of two and three children whose breasts, after nursing, were quite firm.

Breastfeeding will prevent stria from forming. Stria (those crinkly skin marks) come about from broken elastic fibers in the skin. Whether you nurse or not, you will either have them or you won't—again, individual variation. Stria cannot be diminished by rubbing the skin with any known lotion or potion. Plastic surgery may help; nursing will not.

Breastfeeding will keep the baby from being allergic. Certainly there are more babies allergic to cow's milk than to human milk, though occasionally one comes along who cannot tolerate his mother even at this early an age.

Breastfeeding will enlarge breasts that were "too small" before. Alas, I have not found this to be the case, nor have I found anything in the literature to back it up. It seems to be a canard that many doctors keep in circulation. It stems from a time when getting pregnant was the answer to everything. Sure, your breasts, however small, will enlarge during pregnancy—and will stay large during the nursing phase. But once this phase is over, more than likely they will go right back down to where they were—in some instances, even becoming smaller.

Breastfeeding tends to make the mother fat. It is true that a lactating woman needs to take in extra protein and calories. However, she need not gain weight if she takes them in a reasonable fashion. Obviously, cake and candy is not the way to get your calories. Too many women use the excuse of breastfeeding to indulge themselves in all the goodies, since they are convinced they are going to put weight on anyway "for the good of the child." Don't kid yourself.

Breastfeeding precludes going on a diet. Depends what you mean by diet. As stated above, you can't just go around eating all the things that are calculated to get you fat. On the other hand, you can't limit yourself the way you would if you weren't nursing. You have to just use your head and your breasts at the same time.

Breastfeeding depends on a relaxed state of mind to keep the milk flowing. True. A woman who breastfeeds because she is pressured into it is quite likely not to succeed. But successful nursing is quite possible—regardless of the size of the breasts—if the mother is motivated.

Once breastfeeding is started, it has to be carried through until the baby is weaned. Not so. You can always stop if it interferes with your life-style and switch to bottlefeeding.

PREPARED FORMULAS—THE PROPPED BOTTLE

Prepared formulas contain proteins, carbohydrates, and fats so that your baby will have the proper nutritional aids to good growth. Don't push his or her growth. Remember that any bottled formula presents the mother (or aunt, cousin, or grandmother) with the temptation to overfeed. Either don't develop the habit—or break yourself of it—of popping the bottle in the infant's mouth and allowing the child to suck him or herself to sleep. Not only is this bad from the standpoint of providing the infant's satiety mechanism with too much stimulus, so that he or she will fall into the habit of always wanting more, but the teeth will be affected. The propped bottle in the bed allows for reflex sucking even when it isn't needed for nutrition. Such an almost constant exposure to prepared formula just because it's convenient for the mother exposes erupting teeth to relatively high concentrations of carbohydrates, prepared formulas being high in this item. This may set up the conditions for developing such dental problems as enamel subject to decay.

The devilish situation described above as the "propped" bottle is created for two reasons: convenience and the desire that the baby should never be hungry. The prepared formula becomes a sort of magic elixir, one that will prevent the child from crying for the bottle, and one that will allow the mother to feel secure in the knowledge that whenever baby wakes he or she will find food, right at the mouth. It is a juxtaposition of unfortunate beliefs reminding one, somewhat, of the tombs of Egyptian kings, where food was also left to hand so that when the ruler woke in heaven he would have plenty to eat. While there are no records of mummies getting fat on these portions, live babies do. For one thing the constant security derived from the proximity of food is carried throughout life, and the growing child will begin to turn to food as the first line of defense whether for solace, anger, or as a sort of opium against any of life's difficulties. For another, allowing the baby to eat when he or she is not hungry allows the child to develop more fat cells to store this extra food. The young person will have trouble with this kind of new growth later on.

So, while you can certainly bottlefeed your baby if breastfeeding is not convenient to your life-style, and still not have the child get fat, you must bottlefeed, not bottle force. This should not just be looked on as a matter of convenience; it should be done with love. Love is not the providing of food. It is, rather, the thoughtful providing of food. Never, throughout your child's life, will you have the opportunity for control and development of his or her eating habits as you have now. How your child eats later on—what he or she will do with food to hamper or enhance life-style—depends very much on how you train the baby. Right now the baby is all yours, but be assured that this situation will change quickly enough. Don't, if you don't have to, share the child's training at this stage. Let the relatives fume—it will prevent you from having a fretting, fat adolescent. And while there are no guarantees that this sort of feeding will absolutely prevent your child's getting fat, you have, at least, given him or her a good base from which to form a personal eating pattern. You will have nothing to reproach yourself for in future years if your child does end up overweight.

After I gave a lecture on this subject one afternoon, a lady in the audience rose to agree with me. "I never give my baby milk at naptime," she said, "only juice."

Her response showed her heart was in the right place; unfortunately, her information was wanting. I am not speaking strictly of milk. I am speaking as well of juices or any other carbohydrate-containing liquids given in a bottle at naptime or bedtime. A nipple charged with carbohydrates that the baby holds in his mouth as he or she sleeps may well lead to tooth decay (as well as obesity) later on. If you insist that your baby must sleep with a bottle, at least let the bottle be filled with water—plain water, not corn syrup or honey. Even this, as I say, is a bad habit for the mother to get into. Your child may look more comfortable with nipple in mouth, but let's face it: is this really true? Or is it you who is more comfortable because you've seen the picture in so many movies and advertisements? Is it the child's health that is important or your satisfaction with conforming to a mold shaped by the advertisers of a particular product? Food advertising affects all ages. To the food industry both you and your baby represent a market. They want your baby to eat as much as possible so he or she will be big and strong and so they will make money. It has been coming more and more to light that these two relationships do not necessarily go together.

WHAT ABOUT SOLID FOOD?

Too often solid food is "forced" on the baby before he or she is ready for it. By "ready" I don't mean that the baby will not eat it; what I mean is that his or her metabolism is not quite equipped to handle it. A future obese child may be the result.

If you are nursing your baby, it is best that you breastfeed as long as possible—for at least six weeks and, if you can, for three months or longer. When your infant is ready to eat solids, he'll let you know. In fact—and I know that to many of you this will sound somewhat dubious—infants should not be given solid foods until they are old enough to express their wishes in the matter. Giving a two-month-old baby solid food is, according to my belief, tantamount to force-feeding. Unfortunately, pressure from your relatives, friends—and, most especially, the advertising industry, particularly as expressed through television—induces many mothers to start their babies on solid food as early as two months. When I say that solid food should be withheld until the infant expresses a desire for it, I mean until the child can sit with support and indicate whether or not he or she wants to be fed. This generally occurs between the ages of eighteen and twenty-four weeks.

Why all this fuss about solid foods? Well, such food has a direct bearing on whether your child may end up obese or not. Giving the infant solid food too early contributes to overfeeding. It is something like the bottle—baby simply must finish. This, in turn, provides the infant with poor eating habits. He may not yet be of an age to be told that he must eat for the people in China are starving (those poor starving Chinese that are the butt end of a mother's terrible example!), but you can bet your boots that the feeding philosophy is the same.

Studies have shown that no more than 16 percent of the infant's total caloric intake should be supplied by protein. It is very difficult to keep it to less than that in a solid-food situation. Protein comprises 7 percent of the caloric content of human milk. When solid food is added to the diet of breastfed babies, it is best given in the form of high-protein cereal and baby food. The solid food given to infants fed formula or cow's milk should be low in protein, since these items are already quite protein rich.

The introduction of solid food generally starts the weaning period, about the time the infant is six months old. However, recently there has been a move to earlier and earlier introduction of solid foods to the infant. In one U.S. study, 67 percent of one-month-old infants were taking solids; by two months, 96 percent were eating solid foods. And, to make things worse from the standpoint of obese babies, such solids are not generally given as a replacement for formula, but in addition to it. This effectively raises the number of calories the infant is taking in. For what reason? Convenience. The mother's convenience, the advertiser's convenience. And in the long run this convenience carries over to the infant, providing the child with the desire to take in more and more food—a desire that increases as he or she gets older. Other studies reveal that by the age of three months most infants in the United States are eating too much of just about everything. No wonder we have a steadily increasing obese population.

Again, let me state emphatically that far too many parents—you who are reading these pages, perhaps—measure their child's health by how much he or she eats and how much weight is gained. You want your child to be the first one on the block to hit the twenty-pound mark. The first in the suck-the-bottle-dry club. The soonest to eat solid food. Parents tend to take an inordinate pride in the baby sweepstakes. The fact that they may be hurting their baby's future on these stakes doesn't occur to them. Only later, when he or she has become a fat adolescent, do they desperately attempt to change eating habits they have themselves inculcated. It is so much easier to not develop these habits in the first place—though it may put you behind in the one-upmanship baby bragging contests. Be a loser in these contests and win a better future for your child as he or she gets older. More is not always better.

THE PRUDENT INFANT DIET

It does seem to make a difference in later life if certain preventive measures are taken in infancy. What you feed your baby can influence his or her chances of developing obesity, heart attacks, high blood pressure, and diabetes later on. A prudent infant diet, according to Dr. Johan C. Pisacano of the State University of New York at Stony Brook, should be started during the first year of life. Infants should be weaned to such a diet at an early enough age so they will not become addicted to high-fat milk and added salt and sugar. The prudent diet for your child during his or her first year, therefore, would include precooked cereal, skim milk, fresh or cooked fruits or vegetables, fish, a ratio of white to red meat of two to one (a good notion to carry throughout life, in fact), a limited number of eggs, plain yogurt, and a natural gelatin dessert.

On a study done of eighty infants on such prudent diets, only a single child was overweight at the age of three, while sixteen of fifty infants fed standard diets became overweight.

By educating the mother (usually the cook and therefore the tastemaker of the family) to eliminate excess sugar, salt, and fats from an infant's diet, the eating habits of the entire family can be influenced toward better nutrition.

WHAT ABOUT SALTED FOOD?

The daily salt requirement of a healthy baby is small—in fact, human milk has a very low salt content, less than that of tap water in many cities. Cow's milk, in comparison, is quite salty, and many of the commonly used infant formulas are high in salt.

Laboratory investigations of young animals show that brief exposures to a high-salt diet in early life can lead, later on, to all sorts of medical difficulties; while this has not been proved to be the case in humans, there is no reason to believe it could not be the same.

Most salt is introduced to the baby when solid food is started. Why? Because most processed baby foods are salted. Why? Because mother tastes them and mother is used to a certain salt taste in her food. The fact that this is not mother's food but baby's food doesn't occur to most mothers; they assume that their particular taste is how the flavor should be—with the result that the salt content has been reported to exceed that of natural food by as much as five to six times for meat, six to sixty times for vegetables, and in excess of one hundred times for dry cereals.

Now, what does all this mean? Despite one of the more pervasive myths around—that salt is necessary in large amounts for everyone's health—there is no evidence that salting baby food as it is processed at the factory is of any benefit to baby. The notion that the baby has an innate appetite for salt is erroneous. It probably stems from the fact that most adults have an "innate" appetite for salt—no doubt brought about by salted baby foods during their infancy. In most instances, it is likely that the mature infant's kidneys are capable of handling this increased salt intake—but what about the effects of later years? And what about the insatiable appetite for salt that many of us develop as young adults? I can remember in my obese days salting everything even before tasting it. I have seen the same course of action followed by diners at restaurants where the salt flows even faster than the wine. Salt, like sugar, is addictive; it's hard to get rid of the habit once it is formed. And, especially for the child already on the way to being obese from an increased intake of calories, salt in excess is going to compound the problem. So, don't try to supply salt for your new baby. And as far as processed baby foods are concerned, shop around and find those that are the least salted, rather than just choosing those that are most likely to hand or the brand name that happens to be "in" at the time.

WHAT ABOUT THOSE SKIM-MILK FORMULAS?

It is true that skim-milk formulas do tend to promote the growth of fat-free tissue in infants. All well and good—so far. However, this is not the panacea that it may appear to be. It is another example of a logical sequence of thought which, when measured up against practicalities, does not work out quite as it is supposed to. At first instance the logic is impeccable: cut down the calories in a baby's milk so he or she will just take in fewer of them, therefore developing fewer fat cells and not becoming obese. Studies have shown, however, that just the opposite may occur. Infants on such a low-calorie "diet" may become obese when they start to eat solid food.

How does this come about? According to researchers at the University of Iowa College of Medicine, babies on the skim-milk formula do consume fewer calories and gain less weight than babies on regular formula. However, infants who drank a skim-milk formula supplemented with vitamins, safflower oil, and iron grew in length as rapidly as 45 babies who received a commercially prepared formula. All well and good. It seems, however, that the babies who were fed the low-calorie formula drank larger amounts of the liquid during the 56-day period of the study. This study of all of the babies began at 112 days after birth.

The problem lies in the greater amounts that the skim-milk

babies drank. If the feeding of such low-calorie formulas teaches infants to eat until their stomachs feel excessively full, though they may still be taking in fewer calories in toto, a bad eating habit is developed. Those of us who have an obesity problem as adults know that this is precisely the way we eat—until our stomach is full, more often than not, excessively. We, at least, can recognize the problem and try to cut down; the baby will not. Later, when baby begins to take in solid foods—and such foods contain concentrated amounts of calories—he or she may well continue to overeat, following this pattern, which has already been developed, and become fat. In such a case the notion of feeding fewer calories in the formula simply backfires. So, you see, things are not always so simple as they appear. In the case of fat children, they almost never are. The parent who comes to me for a "simple solution" for his or her fat child is whistling in the wind. What must be found is a workable compromise for everyone's taste. As always, the tastes of the individual must play a part. No single answer will serve.

COMMERCIAL VERSUS HOMEMADE BABY FOOD

Are the baby food processors doing anything about reducing the amounts of salt, sugar, and modified starches they have previously been adding to their commercial product? Not only do these items take up a lot of room, displacing nutritious ingredients, but, as I have pointed out, they can result in the infant developing such medical problems as obesity, high blood pressure, and kidney trouble later on.

Well, according to *Consumer Reports,* some changes have been made. The Beech-Nut Company as well as H. J. Heinz announced they were bringing out a line of "natural" baby foods. According to the spokesmen for these companies, all the salt has been taken out of their products, and the number of products to which they have added sugar has been reduced. Gerber, however, at least at this writing, with about 65 to 70 percent of the market, continues to add salt and sugar to many of its baby foods.

But, again according to *Consumer Reports*, even those companies that have modified their product haven't really gone far enough. Here's the way it works out according to figures provided by the companies:

	Number of baby food products	% with added salt	% with added sweeteners	% with modified starches
Beech-Nut	131	0	36	46
Heinz	108	0	33	49
Gerber	152	64	41	44

Then, the labels do not always tell the whole story. Beech-Nut and Heinz, at the time of this writing, are labeling the percentage of added sugar or sweetener; Gerber just lists ingredients in order of prominence. None of the companies uses ingredients such as preservatives, monosodium glutamate, flavor enhancers, artificial flavors, or colors in their baby foods.

MAKING YOUR OWN BABY FOOD

What's the answer then? Is it true that for the mother who wants to provide as proper a nutrition as possible for her child, no matter which way she turns she must compromise her baby's future health? Well, one possible way out of the dilemma is to make your own baby food. It isn't difficult, and you will very likely find it emotionally rewarding. It may not be quite as convenient as buying the commercial variety, but you will know that your infant is being provided for far more properly as far as nutrition is concerned. Homemade baby food need contain no added starch, salt, or sugar. All you need is a grinder. There are several available. *Consumer Reports* lists two: the Happy Baby Food Grinder 500 (Bowland Jacobs Mfg. Co, Spring Valley, IL.) and the similar Sears Baby Food Grinder (cat. no. 17165). Both of these items are plastic and are easy and convenient to use; a moist purée is the result. Of the two, *Consumer Reports* rates the Happy Baby food grinder over the Sears as cleaner to use (the Sears shed bits of metal onto some of the initial food samples—not too nutritious an additive). There may be other grinders in your immediate area that would serve the turn. Certainly you should consider alternatives to what the baby food industry seems to be doing to your infant as far as addicting him or her to their products. Is this a self-serving device to help create an audience for all those TV carbohydrate commercials later on? You can't miss with a captive audience trained from infancy to eat a specific product—no matter what you end up calling it. What's in a name? Obesity, hypertension, kidney disease, psychoses . . .

THE CHUBBY CHILD AND EARLY DIETING

Having come this far and looked over a number of the pros and cons, where do we stand? Is early dieting, though perhaps needful, safe for the developing baby no matter how fat he or she seems to be getting?

Opinion in the medical field is by no means onesided on this point. My feeling is that if your infant does become over-weight—or, worse, obese—something must be done. Obviously—I hope it is obvious—a crash diet is not the answer. Most of the mothers I have spoken to receive very little help on this point from their pediatricians, and many of these mothers, obese themselves, are extremely anxious to prevent their off-spring from following in their footsteps. Yet what do their pediatricians tell them? "Don't worry, he or she will outgrow it." Or, "When she begins menstruating she'll lose." Or, "Try not to feed the child so much."

These are all helpless statements. What does one do for the obese baby? Well, the treatment goal is not really weight reduction, as it is in the adult. That is a rather dangerous game to play with a developing infant. Rather the aim should be to slow down the rate of weight gain to an extent that matches the child's growth pattern more accurately. If you start severely restricting the diet, you may reduce the fat-free body tissues such as protein that will inhibit growth and deplete those energy reserves the child needs to live normally. One thing you can do as a parent that will unequivocally help is to allow your baby as much free movement as possible. Let him wiggle his arms and legs, wag his head, squirm about as much as possible. Some mothers become alarmed when their babies "squiggle about in the crib," thinking something is bothering it. Not so. Physical activity, in infants as in adults (at which time we call it "exercise"), is very important for proper utilization of the food.

In general, the six-month-old period seems to be the critical point at which chubby infants are more likely to become overweight or obese adults than normal or light-weight infants will. This is by no means a 100 percent situation, one researcher finding that weight at this age is predictive of future obesity in close to 40 percent of such children. Of course, if your child is so selected, as far as you are concerned the statistics are 100 percent. However, you should keep in mind that other factors as well as overeating play a part in the development of the chubby child to the chubby adolescent. Such things as the effects of birth weight, rate of weight gain, height, sex, the birth order in relation to brothers or sisters, the competetive environment thus established, breast or formula feeding, social and educational status of the parents—to say nothing of whether or not the parents are obese—all these items add up to tip the scale against the overweight child, who is, so far, taking in on top of this more calories than his body can handle.

It has been assumed by many parents, and many doctors as well, that the tall heavy infant is at less risk of adult obesity than the short heavy one. This, now, does not quite seem to be the case. A recent series of studies showed that the absolute weight gained at six months is the critical variable, quite independent of the length of the child.

What, then, can you as a parent do? The first thing is to recognize the problem. Recognize the problem concerning what you feed your child. Learn as much as you can about nutrition from this and other books on the subject. The higher your educational level regarding this and ancillary subjects, the less chance your child will have of becoming obese, independent of other factors. And, of course, there must be a final return to the subject of your own weight. Your weight status, and that of your partner, shows a striking relationship to whether or not your child will be obese. In one group of children studied, two thirds of all the overweight and obese adults were identifiable by six months of age. The fault, if fault there be, lies not in your child's stars—but in you.

CHILD-SIZE SERVINGS

	2–3 Years	3–6 Years
Milk	6-oz. cup or glass (¾ measuring cup)	6-oz. cup or glass (¾ cup)
Juice	3–4 oz. (⅓–½ cup)	4-oz. glass (½ cup)
Eggs	1 medium	1 medium
Meat	About as much as a cooked meat patty 3″ across, ½″ thick (6–7 patties to 1 lb.)	About as much as a cooked meat patty 3″ across, ½″ thick (6–7 patties to 1 lb.)
Cereal	2 tablespoons cooked, ⅓ cup ready-to-eat kinds	¼ cup cooked, ½ cup ready-to-eat kinds
Bread	½ slice	1 slice
Fruits and Vegetables	½ medium apple, tomato, orange; others, 1–2 tablespoons	½–1 medium apple, tomato, orange; others, 2–4 tablespoons

Source: National Dairy Council.

5

A Helping Hand for the Fat Child

Once your child is old enough to be reasoned with, he or she may be able to understand that obesity, though a difficult problem, is not incurable. This, however, will not make the job of losing weight any easier if your child has already developed poor eating habits. In order for the child to lose weight—and keep it off—it is important that the child have (1) A strong motivation to lose weight, (2) some degree of maturity, and (3) a fairly high tolerance to frustration. This last is most difficult, and a lot of the child's success here will depend on the diet counselor. Overly anxious parents may not only cause the problem to intensify but may dislocate the child's future adjustment to the problem.

THE COMPETITIVE PARENT

Up to the time your child becomes an adolescent—let us say by roughly nine years of age—you, the parent, have pretty much been in control of the food source. This control, which can be exercised stringently at an early age, begins to wane as the child gets older and gets out of the house more and among his or her peers. That is why I have stressed so firmly in preceding chapters the necessity of your exercising this control as effectively as possible while you still had the chance. At adolescence, parental attempts at control, as stated above, can be, at best, useless, at worst, destructive—with all the best will in the world.

Mary M. came to me not long ago. She was ten years old and fat. She had come to the conclusion that she needed to get the weight off quite independently of any parental prodding. However, her mother also had weight to lose, so the two decided to go on one of my weight plans together. Mary M. was most emphatic about seeing me without her mother in the room, a request I was glad to oblige her with, though her mother seemed somewhat disconcerted by it. "After all, Mary," she said, "what have you got to tell the doctor that you can't tell me?" The child's answer was well put. She said that she felt her weight loss was her business—hers and mine—and she wanted to assume the responsibility for it herself. Her mother finally agreed, though reluctantly.

For a while Mary did lose weight. She came to see me separately from her mother—who was also losing weight. Then I began to notice that Mary's weight loss was beginning to slow down. She once asked me if I was telling her mother how she was doing; I said that I could not deny her mother the information if she asked me. In the meantime, the mother, an attractive-looking woman, was losing weight with very little difficulty. As the mother lost, Mary began to gain. The mother stopped asking me how Mary was doing—but Mary began asking me how her mother was doing. Finally Mary gave up. She said she just couldn't compete with her mother, who by now was at normal weight. I suggested that the best thing to do was for Mary to go to another doctor and have her mother stay on my plan. The underlying element of competition Mary developed for her mother's weight loss was sabotaging her own. Yet the mother did not try to counsel Mary; she tried her best to stay neutral. But her body image was something Mary could not stand up against. By changing to another plan and another doctor, one with whom her mother had nothing to do, she managed to take off most of her weight. Today both Mary and her mother are at normal weight—but it was not something they could do together. Certainly in this case any attempt by the parent to counsel the child would have only added to the spirit of competition the child already felt toward the parent.

THE THREE WEIGHT-GAIN PERIODS

The above story demonstrates how great a part the psychological element plays in weight reduction in children. As I will keep saying throughout the course of this book, the problem is not limited to any one element.

At the same time, the nitty-gritty physical putting on of weight does occur at three fairly well-defined points in the child's life. During these periods it is most dangerous for him or her to overeat. One of these times we have already discussed. It is during the intrauterine period—the third trimester, that is, when the mother is in her eighth or ninth month. The mother's overeating at this time will transfer the effect, in many instances, to her unborn child. The second period is during the first two years of life. Again, here, the parent, the mother particularly, has control of how much the child will eat—certainly more so than at the time of the third weight-gain period, the preadolescent period. During all these periods it seems there is a growth in the number of fat cells. If a youngster has this kind of "fat cell" obesity, it can be most difficult to treat. In other words, such children have a large *number* of fat cells as compared to a lower number of them which are simply being enlarged.

THE FAMILY UNIT EXPLORED

What do you do if, not really having been faced with (or having faced) the problem before, you discover you have a fat adolescent or preadolescent on your hands? Remember, a certain percentage of children may become fat during the third weight-gain period, as noted above. This may be the first indication of fatness to come. You should sit down and take stock. Consider the child within the family unit. Remember that every child is an individual—the obese child no less than the normal-weight one. Consider the following points concerning your obese child. What was his or her birth weight? The baby that is heavier at birth tends to have more problems with obesity later on. What is your race and social background? Are you and/or your husband obese? Was this child breastfed when a baby? What about physical activity—not only of the child alone but of the family as a whole? Is physical activity encouraged? And, if so, is this just lip service or does the family indulge in some sport as a family in toto? Skiing is becoming a very popular sport for family togetherness, but it needn't be skiing; any active sport will do. The important thing is for the family, whenever possible, to do it together. That makes it more like the fun it should be rather than as primarily therapy for the fat child. But, other than this group activity, how much reasonable exercise does the overweight child get per day, and can it reasonably be increased? Does the child walk to school or get a ride for a few blocks? What about lunch—does the child buy it in school or bring it from home? What about peer pressures at school? It is absolutely useless for a mother to spend time preparing a reasonable lunch for a child to take to school if the child is simply going to be too embarrassed to eat it, knowing his peers will be eating theirs at the cafeteria. In such a case the child bringing his or her lunch is marking himself out as "different" from his peers; something very few children will want to do. Your child may be telling you emphatically that he or she is eating the lunch you packed, but the chances are at least even that this may not be the case. The child may be buying lunch—or extra food. Should you allow him or her money for this? And, if you do not, will this lead to a disturbed child/parent relationship that will only make the child eat more to spite you?

You will have to devote a considerable amount of your time to mulling these points over. When you have at least isolated these possible reasons for your child's overweight, and you have your own psyche as reasonably set as possible, then it is time to approach the child and have a talk. Within the substance of the family group, that is, with both parents taking part, the child should be encouraged to give his or her views on the subject. You should not lead the child but rather lay the problem out in a sympathetic manner and then ask what he or she proposes to do about it. It is the rare child, in my experience, who, having the situation thus analyzed, will turn around and refuse to do anything about it. In such a case, the parent must try to assume what command of the food activities is possible. Since this is far from total control at this point in the child's age, such a solution is just barely better than nothing.

But, as I say, most children will have recognized the problem for themselves and are probably just waiting to see which way parental concern will manifest itself. Remember, it is not possible to force the child to go on any weight reduction plan. The desire to limit calories, in any manner, must come from the child, and the incentive to continue doing this must come from the diet counselor, whoever this may be. In most successful cases, the counselor is not the parent.

CHECKING WITH YOUR FAMILY DOCTOR

Your family doctor may or may not be the best diet counselor for your child. If he is to take over the job he must have several qualifications. First of all, he must be prepared to devote a lot of time to the situation. Most doctors in general practice of pediatrics are not ready to do this. For another, he must show a genuine interest in his young patient—which includes, of course, delving into all past attempts at losing weight. The most important part of therapy is, of course, motivation. For the parent to say, as all too often they do say to me, "Doctor, you have got to make my child lose weight," is quite a useless remark when I know the child, sitting in quiet rebellion, hasn't the faintest desire in the world to lose weight. What can the family doctor—or indeed any doctor—do in such a case? Likely, nothing at all. It is already a situation that is out of everybody's hands. It has been allowed to develop for too long. What I usually say to any parent who wants their child to lose weight is "Bring the child in to me and let me question the child alone. There is no charge for this, and I make no guarantee I will accept the child as a patient." If, after talking to the child, I find the child uncooperative, I tell the parent, "Let your youngster alone for the present. When he or she is ready and wants to lose weight, then come back and see me and we will talk about it again."

Remember, as an anxious parent seeking immediate relief from the family doctor, treating obesity takes time. The family doctor may not be the one to cope with your child's problem; he may not be able to furnish the proper time. Certainly a quick handful of pills is not the answer. It is just too easy for any doctor to operate on the "parent factor." This, bluntly, means pleasing the parent. All that is involved here is a friendly pat on the child's head, a quick weigh-in, a magic diet list, and maybe a prescription for some pills "that will do the job." There is no such thing as a pill that will do the job. The only pill that will do the job is situated on your child's shoulders. Teaching him or her to use it is the primary job of the diet counselor. For such a counselor you may well require the services of a specialist in the field. Such a doctor, a bariatrician, has been trained in nutrition and obesity. The search for a diet counselor may well lead you to one of these individuals. In any event, the counselor should be a physician. I feel this should be the case when any nutritional problem is being treated, obesity above all. In no case should you trust your child's future health and development to any hands but those of a physician. As I have tried to point out, not all physicians are equally capable of doing the job, but certainly a physician-controled program should be what you finally end up with.

WHAT ABOUT GLANDULAR OBESITY?

I am asked about this all the time, of course. Many parents simply cannot face up to the fact that their child is fat because he or she is being self-indulgent with food. This does not conjure up the sort of picture they want to accept; they would like to blame the child's obesity on a less emotionally charged reason. "I think my son—or daughter—needs thyroid," such a parent will declare at the very first visit. And, in some instances, if this medication is not forthcoming, the parent will march out of the office, child in tow. But I think as a concerned parent you have to understand that the percentage of glandular obesity is very small. As long as the child's height is satisfactory, hypothyroidism is not very likely. The problem is not with the thyroid but somewhat higher. The problem is exogenous obesity, not glandular obesity. One mother I spoke to recently just would not accept that solution. I said that a blood test would have to be done.

"My son just had a blood test," she retorted, triumphantly, "and it came back 'sluggish thyroid.' Now what do you say to that?"

I said that this was not a diagnosis. And she left, still unhappy. But the fact is that the word "sluggish" is meaningless. I am convinced in my own mind that this means that the doctor doing the exam, not the patient's thyroid, is sluggish. What the doctor may be saying is that the thyroid test is equivocal. All that means is that it is probably low normal—but the word normal, not the word low, should be emphasized. Thyroid is a very potent hormone and should not be given indiscriminately to adults, much less children. By insisting your child get it—and some doctors are all too ready to oblige—what you may be doing is adding to, not subtracting from, the child's obesity problem. For adding thyroid does not necessarily increase the body's metabolism. When it may do to a normally functioning thyroid, no matter how low, is suppress the function of the gland, which can have disastrous consequences later on. Do you want to assume the responsibility for this simply because you refuse to face the harsh reality of the situation? I don't!

WHAT ABOUT SURGERY FOR CHILDHOOD OBESITY?

It has been something of a vogue in the past to do all sorts of intestinal bypass procedures. I think that anything like this should be undertaken, if at all, strictly as a last resort. Any surgical candidate should be at least 300 percent over the ideal weight based on height. In no case should you allow your doctor to recommend surgery without a full trial of medical and psychologic therapy. In only a particular instance is surgery perhaps called for, a condition known as the "Pickwickian syndrome." In this condition a tremendous amount of fat is present on the chest itself, leading to the patient's inability to breathe well.

As for the syndrome itself, I'd like to say a few words, however brief, because a little knowledge is a dangerous thing, and I have found more and more mothers coming and telling me that their child may have Pickwickian syndrome. Usually they have picked up a symptom or two in general conversation with a friend and are all too quick to apply the problem, out of sheer anxiety, to their fat child.

The name comes from Dickens. Fat Joe, a character in *The Pickwick Papers*, was a boy who kept falling asleep. He was, as his name implies, very much obese, and he also had trouble breathing. It is especially difficult for individuals like Fat Joe to breathe at night in bed. The excess weight they carry tends to diminish their ability to breathe in a prone position; they keep waking up through the night. In addition, the amount of energy they are forced to use in breathing exhausts them. It is because of this, as well as the disrupted sleep mechanism, that causes such individuals to be so fatigued during the day.

This certainly does *not* mean that all extremely obese individuals have the problem; indeed, a surprising number of them do not. So don't make things worse than they already are by assuming a disease that your child in all likelihood not only doesn't have but will not get. You are already anxious about the problem, don't compound your anxieties.

BEHAVIOR MODIFICATION: THE COST EFFECTIVE THERAPY

My own treatment of both adults and children involves a procedure called "behavior modification." While there are general rules for this type of treatment, there is also sufficient variability to allow for individual variation. It has been proved that behavior modification helps both adults and children lose weight effectively and healthfully—and shows the least tendency to allow the pounds to come back on. Since repeat visits to a nutritionist or dietitian or trained clinician, under a doctor's supervision, is more the routine than expensive prescriptions, health spas, injections, and all the other mystical paraphernalia that seems to go along with weight loss in this country, the treatment is comparatively inexpensive. And, as far as children are concerned, it is something I have been using in my own office for over ten years with very effective results. A report written for the publication *American Journal of Diseases of Children* recently stated: "There is every reason to believe that behavior modification will play an increasingly important part in the treatment of childhood obesity . . . and because about 80 percent of obese children become obese adults, it is important to treat the problem early."

What is behavior modification, exactly, and how can it be used to control childhood obesity?

By analyzing a child's eating habits and using behavior therapy to change the stimuli for eating, to control the very act of eating, and to reinforce certain changes in eating behavior, I have found that many instances—in fact, most instances—of childhood obesity can be treated successfully. It is a technique that can be utilized in the home once a cooperative atmosphere has been achieved between parent and child. It is just about the only effective approach that can be instituted in the home. This does not mean that the child still does not require an outside counselor. But he or she will be seeing this counselor maybe once a week. It is on the days between visits to the counselor that behavior modification in the home can, if properly employed, make a lasting effect, one that will be reinforced by the outside influence. Together, within and without the home, a gradual exercising of control can be established. This control will be erratic at first—after all, what is harder to change than a basic habit pattern?—but, with patience and understanding, eventually the rules of behavior modification will begin to take over. At that point your child need never be fat again.

Here are some of the principles involved:

Practice stimulus control. This involves limiting the accessibility of food. After all, your child can't eat it if it isn't there. True, you can only be responsible for the home environment, but at least you have that much under your control. Remember, if it's there he or she will probably eat it. Not only should food be eliminated from the home environment, or at least its easy accessibility, but all cues that signal eating behavior should be blunted. The TV is an important element here. Food (snacks) and TV must be separated. Instead, new cues should be developed that have nothing to do with food. In order to reduce the number of food-reminding stimuli around the home, try to have the child eat only when truly hungry and only at one place in the house, do not use food as a reward mechanism, and discourage eating in bed.

Slow the rate of eating. Under no circumstances should the child be permitted to speed through a meal. This must be held to even if the child is late for school. He will simply have to get up earlier. He must learn to chew food, not bolt it. Only in that way will he be able to acquire enough oral satiation not to want another meal as soon as he is finished gobbling down this one.

Reward weight loss and behavioral changes. Children like and expect rewards when they have done something well. Don't be ashamed to tell the child he has done well—and give him some tangible account of it. He should be rewarded promptly for any small behavioral changes as well as for weight loss itself. Such rewards as toys, money, extra TV viewing time, and any other special events come in very handy. Of course, the most popular rewards that parents ordinarily use—those involving food (ice cream, cookies, candy)—are not only out but shouldn't even be in the house, much less mentioned.

Reinforce the child's self-image. The obese child has a very poor picture of himself, no matter how he may attempt to make light of it. This self-image should be restructured. No negative statements should be tolerated. Gently but firmly, the child must be given a more positive self-image. Such remarks as "I let the kids use me as second base" or "I don't care if the other kids make fun of me—at least they notice me" are poor substitutes for present longings of companionship and may well develop into psychoses later on in life.

Change the act of eating. Eating, if possible, should be done in the same place each time. The best place is usually kitchen or dining room. The bedroom is a bad place to eat. The habit pattern of eating in bed becomes, in itself, a luxury, and whenever the child goes to bed he will begin to associate this act with food—as many adults do. In front of the TV is not a good place to eat. In fact, eating should be done as a solitary act. No other act should accompany it. Watching TV or reading a book or playing with toys or having an argument—all of these activities detract from the act of eating, make it secondary to something else. We've all had the experience of going into a store where background music is playing. We may be in the store for an hour making a purchase, the music playing all the while. But when we leave can we remember one tune we've heard? No— because the music was part of the background. When food becomes part of the background of other things, it, too, becomes an unthinking activity.

Slow down the act of eating. The act of eating slowly in itself can be aided by putting knife and fork on the table in between bites. Somehow when we hold our eating utensils in our hands we feel inclined to keep them in use—and so we take bites of food fairly rapidly. Having to pick up and lay down our utensils helps slow down the eating time. Children are very good at bolting their food. Unfortunately, eating fast leads to a more rapid return of hunger, since the mouth has not been satisfied. Better by far to eat slowly.

Reduce emotional stress. In other words, get off the kid's back. One way to make your kids eat more is to keep harping on the subject, keep denigrating them—especially in front of other people. I've had patients do this to their children in the office in front of me. In at least one instance the child was a patient. The mother kept complaining so about how "bad" he had been during the week that I felt like eating myself out of spite. Sure you want to take an interest in your children's health—but one thing they'll quickly get fed up with is constant nagging.

Another type of emotional stress that leads to eating is boredom. While I don't expect you to be a constant provider of entertainment for your children, it's a good idea to get them interested in some hobby so they can entertain themselves as they grow older. This can be sports or dance, stamp collecting or pottery making. But give them enough of an introduction to several outlets for their creative energy to keep boredom to a minimum. Eating for the sake of eating is not a good hobby.

In this manner, by analyzing your child's eating habits you can use behavior therapy to change the stimuli for eating, control the act of eating, and reinforce changes in eating behavior. This will help the child's weekly visits to the counselor.

WHAT ABOUT EXERCISE?

No question but that exercise is a very important part of the overall view here. I mention exercise for the fat adolescent especially, since there has been quite a lot of comment in medical circles disputing its effectiveness. It has been shown with movies, for example, that the obese child moves more slowly than the lean one at whatever he or she is doing—whether it is swimming or playing basketball or just walking. The obese youngster, moving slower, will not burn up the amount of calories that a lean youngster will. Getting such a slow-moving individual to participate in any form of exercise can in itself be an exercise in frustration. You can't just say, "Joseph, go out and exercise." Maybe you do say it—but will Joseph do it? What you have to provide are some very definite things for the exerciser to do. Walking, as I have said in all my books, whether for child or adult, is an excellent activity for burning calories. Walking an hour a day—briskly—burns away a lot of food. For children, have them pick out a spot, maybe twenty minutes or half an hour away from home, to walk to and back, and work a reward system into the plan so it won't become "work." Anything a child considers "work" is going to develop into a "no show" condition sooner or later. Whatever you do, especially for the preadolescent or beginning adolescent child, keeping it simple is the most effective approach.

Let's not forget that the obese child really would much rather not be obese. Therefore, he or she will try. They will try to oblige, try to follow directions, try to compete whether on the basketball court or the dance floor. But what happens is that the competition just becomes too much for them, and pretty soon, disheartened, they are just standing around watching, not getting involved. Schools, with all their emphasis on exercise, still pay more lip service to it—where the obese child is concerned—than anything else.

I have found that an exercise group with all fat kids works out much better than one mixing the fat with the lean. Somebody has to hit the baseball, run the bases, hit the volley ball over the net. In a group of obese children, this of necessity has to be an obese child. For any one of them to do it makes it a triumph, in a way, for all of them. Conversely, in a thin/obese group, every time an obese child is defeated, it is a defeat for them all.

One way to get a group of obese kids organized is at your pediatrician's office. He certainly will know of more than one. It would be worth your while as a parent to try to get a group like this going for a sport/exercise program. Rather than have to hunt up applicants, chances are you will have more than you can handle.

6

Face to Face: The Fat Kid's Chapter

Up to now I've been pretty much talking to your parents. For several reasons. For one, up to now you haven't really been all that interested. Perhaps you haven't been terribly involved with the problem, even though it is yours. But you've been home, among your family, and you've allowed things to take their course. Or courses. Everything, as they say, from soup to nuts.

Now what's driving you nuts is your weight. Suddenly it's become a real drag. You aren't happy about it; trying to make the best of it is, at best, a fairly defeating experience. It's next to impossible to discuss it with your parents, really, unless you have a very unusual household. They're probably too close to you to be objective enough to help. Perhaps, you feel, they don't want to help. Many parents aren't terribly interested in an overweight kid; they figure the weight came on by itself, it will go off by itself. So there you are, as I've said, drifting. Or, as you may think, sinking—under your own weight. What can you do about it? Let's talk about it face to face. Just you and me.

IT'S REALLY YOUR PROBLEM

What you can do about it is start using your head. Not the bottom portion—you already use that part quite well. I'm talking about the top portion, the part you use later on to regret what you've used the bottom part for. You have to use your head, not your feet, to take a stand against the creeping tide of fat that is otherwise really going to flood you. Remember that more than 60 percent of children who are overweight at four years of age become overweight adults. It has been estimated that if childhood-onset obese persons have not slimmed down by the end of adolescence, the odds against their doing so as adults are 28 to 1. So the time is now. And the first thing you have to consider is that this problem won't go away by itself. And it won't go away at all overnight. It's going to take a long time to get rid of the weight you are carrying. That's not fun to consider, but even less fun to consider is the fact that if you don't do something about it now, you'll get fatter.

A SELF-MANAGEMENT APPROACH

The situation, however, is far from hopeless. You've just got to rearrange a few of your ideas, for a start. We're going to talk about "pre-dieting"—getting the fat off now, while it's still easy, before you become an adult and have to go on a real diet. You are going to be the doctor and the patient. I'll help you be the doctor. You have to select the right patient attitude.

In my office I counsel obese adolescents like you about how to take a self-management approach to this problem. I can talk to you pretty much face to face as I talk to them. I can't see you, of course, but I assume since you are reading this chapter that you are fat, that you need help. You need help to lose weight, and losing weight can only come about, really, by selecting what you eat so you don't continue to feed your obesity. Here are some of the things you will want to do to self-manage this nasty situation effectively. They aren't difficult to do, but they are difficult to keep in mind. If you will just read them through and consider each point as a separate little exercise to be done each day—right from the beginning—you will find yourself looking and feeling better almost immediately. Part of this feeling better is the knowledge that you are doing something to help yourself, that you are relying on your own strength, not on the strength of your parents. Their strength will not be able to help you in this endeavor.

Give yourself a really good look. The best way to get a really good look at yourself is to do it with a camera. Have someone take your picture. Best results are obtained by wearing shorts and a tee-shirt for your picture. Don't worry about breaking the camera; what you want to do is to break the spell of fatness. Give your picture a really good going over. You needn't show it to anyone else; in fact, it's better if you don't. The idea behind taking your picture, of course, is to get all of yourself under your eye, to take what is called an inventory of the problem. It's also a good idea to continue taking your picture all through your weight loss, an interval of every 15 or 20 pounds being generally effective. This will show you what sort of progress you are making. Of course you want to see progress, since losing weight involves a lot of hard work, and the only way to really see how much improvement you are making is to look at yourself through the impersonal eye of the camera.

In my office I take these pictures and mount them on a stiff sheet of paper in the order in which they are taken. I write the date under each one and also the weight. You should do the same. In this way you will not only have an initial overall view of the problem, you will have a precise measure of your success in the change in how you look. Otherwise, you won't really be able to tell. Oh, you'll feel the difference in your clothes, of course, but the idea of changing from one person to another is more dramatically shown in pictures of the process as it is occurring.

Make your appearance something to be proud of. Many young people come to me as patients looking pretty scruffy, to put it frankly. The idea seems to be they look pretty lousy, anyway, being fat, so what is the use in trying to look any different in their choice of wardrobe, hairstyle, or grooming in general? Well, it makes a very big difference. For one thing, you feel better when you look as well as you can. When you present as good an appearance as you can, you will always be trying to improve that appearance. When your outward appearance is disheveled, what you are really saying is that you don't care how you look. It's a kind of giving up. I don't want you to give up anything except the foods that are making you fat. You should place a high value on your appearance even if you feel your fat is against you. As you see your appearance begin to change—even if your weight hasn't yet begun to do so—it will encourage you to make your entire profile change. It is important that you have something to feel good about.

It's awfully easy to give up. It isn't nearly as easy to look up. Yet that is what I'm telling you to do. You have to look up to yourself, to be the best that you can be in outward as well as inward presentation. If you look like a failure, you will be able more easily to convince yourself that you are one. It's really as easy to be a success as a failure. All it takes is being able to first dress the part. It is always interesting to me to see the difference in people—young as well as old—as they start to lose weight. They begin to buy clothes, while before they made do with hand-me-downs; they begin to groom themselves, while before they slopped around; they begin to have self-respect, while before they had only a dismal sense of frustration. You can start your weight loss program right away by getting yourself off your back. That way you'll be able to look yourself in the face and recognize the person you want to be.

Don't call yourself names. "I cheated this week." "I ate garbage." "I was really bad yesterday." "Doctor, all I did was stuff myself with junk." "I really blew it. Guess I'm really no good."

All the above are phrases of self-reproach I hear pretty regularly at Weight Loss Control. Read them again. Does something strike you about them? They are all more than excuses—there's nothing wrong, incidentally, with a good excuse—they are self-reproaches, name calling. Take number one. Did you "cheat"? That means that you are a cheat. A cheat is generally looked down on, someone who is pretty much not wanted, a person to be despised. Isn't that a little strong just for eating some food that wasn't on your plan for the day? What these excuse–name callings do is make the person using them overreact. If you have settled the matter that you are a cheat, that you eat garbage, that you really are no good, where is there to go from there except further down? You can't do this to yourself. Don't let anyone else do it to you. It's a way of saying to yourself, "What's the use?" Yet, if you really felt that way you wouldn't bother feeling bad about being fat; you'd be fat and enjoy it. In this case you wouldn't be reading this book anyway. You'd be reading a cookbook. *How to Cook Your Own Goose* is the name of this cookbook—and chances are you already know it by heart. Calling yourself names in the form of these excuses only gives you more reasons to eat. Stop it right now. Take a deep breath and say to yourself, "I will do the very best I can. If that is only being on my plan 70 percent, that is still better than 50 percent, which is better than 30, which is better than 20, which is better than not at all." And that's the way you must think.

Set reasonable goals for yourself. Let's face it—you aren't going to change from craving Burger Kings with French fries to eating raw vegetables right off the bat. Nor, in fact, do you have to ever make this kind of turnabout. What you have to consider is making changes slowly. One change per week is a very good rate of speed. Try to work a change in some aspect of your eating procedure on a weekly basis—and, of course, maintain it as you add another and another. Such things as your food habits, your eating style, your positive thinking about yourself and your problem, your self-assertiveness are all mental exercises that can be reviewed and reinforced each week as you keep building them up. Add to these the physical portions of your weight-loss plan, such as what you eat and how you exercise. It is the combination of all these factors that will start slimming you down.

Keep your family informed. Your family is worried about you. Sometimes parents can be more bother to you in trying to help, than if they were dead set against your making any progress. But that's part of the interrelationship of many families, not just yours. Be patient with your parents. They have their own anxieties about you—which are, admittedly, not always constructive. You should at least try to discuss with them what you are doing and the measure of success you are achieving. Your visits to your doctor can be accomplished by you, without your parents being present, but you probably would feel bad if they showed no interest at all. Make sure your parents know that you are trying in your own way to succeed. That's the only way you *can* succeed. If this has caused a family strain, talk to your doctor and see if he can help straighten things out. What is most important to remember is that losing weight is a very personal, very individual concern. But it is also the concern of your parents; they are entitled to help you. While the line between helping and interfering isn't always clearly marked, patience on both parts will help.

WHAT ABOUT WILLPOWER?

You may not realize it, but kids have more willpower than adults. Kids can do almost anything they set their mind to. Why? For one thing, unlike adults, you have fewer past failures to contend with. A lot of adult frustrations are all mixed up with past wrong turnings and emotional tangles. You can start out pretty much with a clean slate. Also, you have a fresh new body to order around, one that hasn't been subjected to the stresses and strains of a hundred previous "diets," as is the case with the average fat adult. You may even be making your first real attempt at this point to lose weight—and if you do it correctly you'll be astonished to find how easy it is, how much willpower you really have.

It is this willpower that, if it does nothing else, will get you to the doctor every week for that all-important office visit. It is this willpower that makes you keep an eye on yourself and remember to note any deviation from your food plan. This kind of watching over yourself can give you a very secure feeling. After all, who is better qualified to watch over you than you?

HOW FAST CAN YOU LOSE?

You have to understand that there is no way every person loses weight at the same rate of speed. However, on a general diet (more specific ones will follow in the next chapter), you can lose more rapidly than you put on the weight. But let's be honest with one another. Don't look for total success. Remember that you are growing, and your goal weight will change because of that.

A typical diet may include egg and toast or cereal for breakfast; a sandwich or soup for lunch; a low-calorie soda or grape-fruit or cantaloupe or pear for afternoon snack, and meat and salad and some vegetables for dinner. In addition, you may have a snack in the evening. With all of this, plus your will-power, in the first three months you can lose about 20 percent of your fat, and in six months you can get close to 50 percent of it off.

But don't let eating be a chore, a punishment because you feel you are substituting "food medicine" for food. All food is good; don't put yourself into a disciplinary situation with it. Eating should be done with a contented mind in pleasant sur-roundings. It doesn't have to be fun, however. Confusing eating with fun only makes you want to eat more—just for the fun of it.

DO YOU KNOW WHAT HUNGER IS?

You can't learn what hunger is at too early an age. You may not be able to grasp all the concepts associated with true hunger yet, but as you grow older you will begin to find many of them quite obvious. Hunger is the message your stomach and your mouth send to your brain when they feel the need to take in food. Any kind of food will satisfy your stomach, since it has no taste buds and doesn't require delicacies. Your stomach only knows if it is full or empty. Your mouth is somewhat more picky, since you do have taste buds in your mouth to help you choose just the kinds of foods that you like. Sometimes, often, these foods you like are what help make you fat. Yet, by taking in other foods that will not make you fat, yet that will quell the hunger in your stomach, you can eat, be comfortable, and even lose weight. The problem is obviously in satisfying true hunger, not in merely catering to appetite or social occasion!

The ability to make this distinction between hunger and ap-petite is essential. I will be showing you in this book how to keep your options open so you will be able to satisfy true hun-ger and not feel deprived, yet still be able to get those fif-teen- to twenty-pound pictures taken. You must remember that hunger is a state of the body, and as such it must be satisfied.

Even if you manage to overlook hunger to the point that it diminishes after a while and seems to go away, it can come back, stronger than before. At this time you may get so hungry that you just eat whatever is at hand. So you are just fooling yourself. A common remark made to me is, "Oh, I eat nothing all day, but at night I gorge myself." Well, what's so good about that? In fact, nothing. It is, in fact, better to eat through the day, when hunger strikes, rather than put it off until night when you pile in the food all at once, thereby giving yourself both indigestion and a guilty conscience.

APPETITE IS NOT HUNGER

If hunger, as I have said, is a state of the body, appetite is a state of the mind. But don't be fooled by that; that doesn't make it any the less real. Hunger is the body calling for food; appetite is your taste for the kind of food you provide your body with. You have to learn to feed your hunger, not your appetite. If your taste is strictly for so-called "junk foods"—refined, processed, "empty calorie" foods such as sweetened sodas, cookies, cake, candy, ice cream, and so forth—you will be adding pounds to your body by feeding your appetite. But, you say, I really have a sweet tooth; I crave sweets. You've probably heard adults say this. Yet you can satisfy this sweet tooth with fruits rather than cake or candy. That way you get to feed your appetite *and* your hunger. In many societies this is just what people do. In this country we are the prey of the manufacturers of sugared goods who have taught our appetites to respond to their products rather than natural items. But it won't be long before you can convert your appetite into the proper channels and start losing weight with it rather than gaining. This book will help you do just that.

7
Ensuring
Success

Children grow rapidly, and because of this their energy and protein needs are high. These kids are burning a lot of calories, and they tend to eat. If the amount of energy they take in in the form of foods, especially carbohydrates, is balanced out by the energy they spend—in sports, exercise, or general activity—then adolescents can eat pretty much at their own dictates. Where the obese adolescent is concerned, however, it is alarmingly evident that more energy is going in than is coming out. The child becomes fatter and fatter; indeed, obesity is prevalent among this age group. The children who are overweight are discriminated against by their peers who do not have the problem. As we know, children can be very cruel. Such "different" children become isolated, depressed, bored—and eat even more. Which compounds the problem all around.

A BASIC REDUCING PLAN

Any reducing plan must, of course, involve reducing the food intake of the fat child, but this must be done carefully. It is good where possible to try to match the needs, foodwise and psychologically, of the individual child. Such individuality is not possible in a book. I must therefore provide a general guide that can be adapted to the needs of a specific child. It must be kept in mind that severe restriction of energy foods may mean that the child's body will use protein foods for energy instead of for building body tissue. This can lead to interference with the growth mechanism.

At the same time, for the the obese adolescent who is becoming more and more bogged down with his own fat, something fairly radical must be done.

Weight reduction for the overweight child is best accomplished by restricting those foods rich in calories but in little else. The high fat and high carbohydrate foods are first in line here. Whether the fat child is best treated in a group so as to get the maximum support from others like him- or herself or individually in a "head to head" confrontation with a counselor is best determined by the principals involved. I personally favor the individual approach. It isn't easy to give up those well-loved cookies, cakes, and candies here and now to improve an image the circumstances of which will take place a ways down the road. Yet, of course, it must be done if anything at all is to be accomplished.

VITAMINS AND MINERALS

Due to the demands of growth, vitamin requirements are increased for all adolescents, and no weight reduction program should take place without including a sufficient supply of vitamins. In general, adolescents in this country tend to undersupply themselves with the several vitamins their bodies require. It has been calculated that they often take as little as 50 percent of certain of the required vitamins. This can lead to anemia and stunted growth. A deficiency in vitamin B_6 is also prevalent, leading to the impaired ability of the body to use dietary protein.

As for minerals, the most likely to be skimped by the adolescent are calcium, iron, and zinc, all of them needed in increased amounts during this blazing period of growth. Calcium is necessary for normal skeletal growth, zinc and iron for both skeletal and muscle growth. Iron is essential for the extra amounts of blood being produced to keep pace with the fast-growing tissue of the body. In short, the faster anyone grows, the more of these items—especially calcium—he needs. And it seems to be calcium in particular that the modern adolescent is cutting out. Most of these kids drink little or no milk and eat few dairy products. The "junk food" syndrome is the worst offender, but processed foods and even increased meat intake play a part in limiting the amount of calcium the body can absorb. So calcium is definitely indicated as a supplement while the obese adolescent is on a weight-control program.

Iron can also be a problem. It has been calculated that between 5 and 15 percent of American adolescents are anemic. Boys, especially, require more iron than girls because of their greater muscle mass (though girls tend to make up for this by losing iron with their menstrual flow). Iron is most easily absorbed from meat but it can be gotten as well from plant sources such as beans and green vegetables. Beans are not usually on a dietary menu. Fortunately iron, like calcium, can be given as a supplement.

The case for zinc is somewhat more to the fore these days than formerly. This trace mineral seems to have something to do with growth and sexual maturation. Many adolescents consume far less of this mineral than they should, a fact especially true of girls, who often take in less than half of what has been calculated as the basic allowance. Zinc is contained in meat, seafood, eggs, and milk. In general, vegetables contain little zinc, and adolescents who are on a vegetarian diet should be certain to get their zinc as a supplement.

In short, supplementation is necessary at this very important time of life. While cutting down on the fat adolescent's food consumption, one doesn't want to cut down on the required substances described above. It is easy enough to supply them, minus the calories, in pill form. There are children who will not take pills. It must be explained to them that these pills are necessary to help keep them in good health and that any diet plan that will be successful in having them lose weight must rely on the outside supplementation of elements that would otherwise be missing in the diet.

THE STUFF 'N' STARVE SYNDROME

Perhaps you've never heard it referred to as such. First you eat too much, then you desperately try to eat nothing at all to make up for it. When an adolescent tries this type of activity, results can be most unfortunate. For one thing, the type of behavior is totally undisciplined and results in extreme swings of mood and conduct; for another, the depletion of necessary nutrients during the "starve" phase is scarcely made up for in the "stuffing" phase, which consists mostly of a carbohydrate orgy. This "crime and punishment" reaction is to be deplored in the adult, but in children it should be avoided altogether.

LET'S TALK ABOUT SNACKS AND JUNK FOOD

A recent Gallup Youth Survey revealed that American teenagers are not the junk food addicts everyone seems to assume. At the same time, there is no doubt that the predilection for pizza and spaghetti carries on from adolescence through the teen years and into adulthood. But is "junk food" really "junk"? Like most other things, no harm comes from junk foods if they are not carried to excess. I permit certain of my patients who are fat adolescents an occasional cheeseburger—and even French fries and a milkshake—since this allows them to be on a level with their peers. Certainly this cannot be an everyday occurrence, but once in a while, if the child is doing well with his weight, he may be allowed such a "fast food" regimen. There are ways, of course, of making the cheeseburger less caloric, and so far as the French fries are concerned, the most important thing to watch is the salt—and the ketchup, which contains more sugar than one might suppose. The challenge here, as far as the fat adolescent is concerned, is to try to give him or her something that fits more with his or her lifestyle—making the foods more palatable and tasty than might be expected on the ordinary "diet." Even allowing the adolescent this "splurge" once a week I find does no harm, as my patients continue to lose weight—provided such splurges are, indeed, limited.

Snacks are another matter. Since snack food is usually a packaged, fast-food meal, it tends in some kids to replace a conventional meal. There seems to be an innate relationship between snack foods and "soda"—and not the low-calorie variety. Unfortunately many, if not all, of the snack foods preferred by adolescents are without any redeeming value. While popcorn, plain and without salt, has some vitamins and minerals in it, one might reasonably try to substitute this for the sugar-coated, high calorie "Crackerjack" type of snack. And popcorn is, of course, a good source of fiber. But try to get any self-respecting adolescent to eat plain, unsalted popcorn. I don't think it is possible. And, once it is covered with salt and butter, popcorn will certainly make a kid pop!

CAUSES FOR FAILURE

Let's look at the problem pessimistically, just for a moment, and then go on an upswing from there. I want to mention why kids fail. It isn't all their fault. Sure, some of the causes are lack of motivation, but a lot of it is lack of parental support; over-emphasis on parental guidance (the nag factor); setting of unrealistic goals, by both parent and kid; unrealistic assumptions of daily weight loss. Then there are the friends and neighbors who "sabotage" the kid's diet by offering goodies that aren't on it and then denying they've done it when you ask them.

There is also the factor of "sticking'-to-it-iveness." Attention is drawn away from diets by social events, a national disaster, the common cold, a vacation. Once the attention span is so dismissed, it is hard to regain. Worse, the diet is itself blamed for this lapse, and many individuals proceed to take revenge on it for its broken promises by eating like mad. I think you must keep in mind that while you and the kids may go on a vacation from dieting, your fat cells never stop packing in the food. They never go on vacation.

HOW THIS METHOD WORKS

Our calories will be derived from all the necessary food substances such as proteins, fats, and carbohydrates. Remember that protein is responsible for building and maintaining the body; fats and carbohydrates are burned to provide energy. It is the fats and carbohydrates that are stored by the body as fat. Keep in mind a simple parallel as far as calories are concerned: one oatmeal cookie (about a hundred calories) eaten daily will add ten pounds in just a year. How fast it goes down—and how surprisingly hard it is to get off! In point of fact, the usual difference between "normal" weight and overweight—even obesity—amounts to just those few extra calories per day spread over a period of time.

Remember, also, that this is not a "miracle" plan. Miracle plan results come and go. Fat is just not meant to be lost rapidly. By "rapidly" I mean as fast as *you* want it to go. A reasonable schedule for weight loss in children may run a pound every three days. Believe me, that is fast enough. Of course, changes in body water balance may result in the loss of quite a few additional pounds during the first week—or even in the first few days. This is a "bonus" weight loss that, while welcome, must not influence the mind of the child to expect such a loss on a continuing basis. It happens all too often that just such a situation occurs. "I'm so thrilled for little Johnny," a mother will tell me. "He was only on your plan for three days and he already lost five pounds." I tell such a parent that this loss will not—can not—continue, and the usual response is, "Oh, I know that." Unfortunately the following week she will report in a disappointed tone, "Oh Johnny only lost two pounds this week." Her disappointed tone carries over to the child, who begins to feel guilty, then disgusted, then desperate—and then gives up. So don't let the initial weight loss get your hopes up so that they are out of line.

As for some of the specific foods, it is a good idea to give poultry and fish an even break with beef and pork. In fact, I like to overemphasize fish and fowl. For some reason the All-American dish of red meat and salad has become the ideal to many people. If a lot of meat is being eaten, it may be the proper time to begin varying what you buy and, as the cook for the family, what you prepare. As far as the meat servings are concerned, be sure to trim away all visible fat—reasonably—and, as far as oils are concerned, rely very little on those from animal sources. Liquid vegetable oils are fine for cooking. In cooking, it is desirable to broil and/or roast meat rather than fry it. Frying is never a terribly good way to prepare food; a little oil goes a long way, as far as I am concerned.

For vegetables, give steamed ones preference over boiled. It is better to buy any fresh or frozen foods rather than canned. Most people automatically take advantage of the season to lay in provisions of fresh fruits and vegetables, but, to my surprise, many of my patients "do not bother." It is a very good idea "to bother." Children, especially, will not go out and buy a piece of fresh fruit, preferring any of the competitive "junk food" items. In order for them to eat nutritious food, it has to be around. So keep it around.

Always read labels. Sometimes, granted they don't tell you very much. But once you get into the label-reading habit, you will be astonished to discover how much you can learn about foods—and how much of the "food" on the market that you may have been buying is nothing more than a collection of chemicals, attractively packaged for your eye, but having little enough to do with the nutrition needs of your family.

As for salt, that ancient enemy of the fat person, use it very sparingly in cooking. Let your family add their own at table, if need be. The fat child, of course, should be taught to add very little, if any, salt to his or her food. Most people do not realize (and many will not be taught) that salt, like sugar, can be addictive.

As far as sugar is concerned, of course, restrict to a minimum all the sugared, "sweet-tooth" items. The fruit you will have in the house should suffice to keep any "sweet-tooth" in line. Your child should learn to depend on fruit rather than seeking candy; this is easiest to teach before the child is beginning to spend more time with his peers than at home. Always discredit the notion, promulgated by visitors, in-laws, and others, that a piece of candy is a "treat." One such "treat", if it establishes a lifelong craving, can require a long series of "treatments."

If you are eating out, there is no reason the fat child cannot go along with you. You do not want to make him or her feel different from yourself or any of the other children in the family who may not have his or her problem. As I keep repeating, the fat child already feels "different" enough. As a former fat child myself, I can remember the sinking feeling of humiliation that always came over me when I had to eat foods that were different from everyone else's because "You don't want to stay fat, do you?" I recall I would willingly have stayed fat if only to avoid the question—always asked in company—and the taste-less food substituted for the goodies everyone else seemed to be indulging in.

What you, as the parent, can do when eating out is to study the menu carefully and ask questions of the waiter. Ask as though the situation applies to yourself, not to any of your children or to anyone else at the table. But don't be ashamed to ask—demand, even—that the food be served a certain way. I recall recently being present at a dinner party where a famous member of royalty was present. I was seated two tables away, but I could hear her giving strict orders to the waiter on how the food was to be prepared for one of the individuals at her table—a young man, as it happened. If she could do it, and not think it too much trouble, why shouldn't you? Never allow the waiter in a restaurant to bully you—if only by his demeanor. And don't carry with you the notion that since "going out" is a treat, the food served to the fat child has to be a treat as well—that is, something not on his diet plan. All of this is what I refer to when I tell you that in order to diet successfully or teach someone else how to, you first have to get the fat out of your head and learn to think nutritionally.

PORTIONING OUT FOOD

It's not hard for parent and child to quickly develop a "food measurement" sense—if you both really want to, that is. First thing to learn is the "hand weight" of a measuring cup; fill such a measuring cup with one cup of any food. Then pour the food from the measuring cup onto a plate. This will give both "hand sense" and "sight sense" of just how much food a measuring cup holds and how much it weighs. Do the same with half a cup, then a cup of various substances. Do the same with a tablespoon; get to know how much salad dressing, for instance, a tablespoon holds. Once you understand this, pour a table-spoon of salad dressing over some lettuce to see how much surface it will cover. Let your child do these little experiments with you; for the fat child to begin to develop a food measurement sense is extremely important. As far as salad dressing is concerned when you are eating out, it is best to request a plain salad and add your own dressing—vinegar and oil or just plain lemon or lime juice are the best choices. Don't accept the word of the restaurant that their salad dressing "doesn't have many calories." The waiter in the restaurant only tells you what you are willing to hear.

The development of a firm concept for meat portions is equally important. I don't want either you or your child to be weighing things. Weighing food is the quickest way I know to get fed up with any diet. I recall when I was a fat child my parents were constantly weighing portions of food. When the portion was too light, I added more, not wanting to be cheated of my rightful share. When the portion was too much, I would eat the excess. I felt quite virtuous upon arriving at the determined weight to put that on my plate and "limit" myself to it.

Determining a ·concept for meat portions can start in the market. Handle, and let your child handle, various weights of meat, poultry, and the like. The determination of a pound portion can be taken as a measure to go to the concept of half a pound and a quarter pound. A bird in the hand is quite literally worth two in the bush—especially when you begin to get the notion of just what various portions of that bird weigh. You can make quite a game of this "portion concept" with your child. But it isn't all a game, it is deadly serious—and behind the amiability of this sort of experimenting is the harsh reality of learning just how much food one is really taking in. Once this concept is developed, both for liquids and solids, your child cannot ever say, truthfully, "I really didn't eat much," when he or she knows pretty much to the ounce what he did eat. This is a fairly sophisticated approach—but if it is employed early in the training of the child, it will quickly become second nature. The child won't be able to fool him- or herself, or you.

At this point it may be a good idea to present the standard table of weights and measures so that you and your child will know precisely what things weigh in both the American and metric systems. Somehow one can never find this table when one wants to lay one's hands on it:

WEIGHTS AND MEASURES

1 pound (16 ounces) = 453 grams
½ pound (8 ounces) = 227 grams
¼ pound (4 ounces) = 113 grams
1 ounce = 28 grams
1 quart = 4 cups
1 pint = 2 cups
1 cup = ½ pint
1 cup = 8 fluid ounces
1 tablespoon = 3 teaspoons

Tables are fine in their purely arbitrary sense; however, one doesn't eat tables, one eats on them. It is critical, therefore, that you translate these weights and measures into hand sense and eye sense, as we have prescribed. As far as losing weight is concerned, this is the most important exercise either you or your child will do.

SOME FOOD FOR THOUGHT

Here are some tips for modifying your child's eating habits. One thing you don't want to do is to try to change all his or her habits at one time. You are best to seek change in gently modifying one or at most two habits at a time. Don't be discouraged if you don't see steady progress; we all regress at times. These tips are best used as a flexible guide, not as rigid rules to be sworn to. You don't want the child to rebel—an all-too-common occurrence. Some of these tips are meant for you, the parents. Remember that a lot of your child's overeating may be your fault. Again, I don't bring this up to give you guilt feelings. I simply want you to understand that behavior modification applies to adults as well as to kids. Let's look at some of these ways parents can help.

1. Don't prepare too much food. If you are the cook in the family, cook only the amount of food you think each member should eat. Avoiding "leftovers" will prevent the eating of same. Your child can't eat what isn't there.

2. *Place the fat child's food on a slightly smaller plate.* Obviously—I hope it's obvious—this can't be carried to extremes. You don't want everyone else eating from dinner plates and the fat child nibbling from a saucer. But within the bounds of reason and kindness, the thing should be done. This, of course, gives the eye sense a bit of a fraudulent impression, the smaller plate presents a larger portion of food. Try the experiment yourself if you don't believe it. Take a serving plate and put on it a standard portion of food for yourself. It doesn't look like much, does it? Those empty portions make the food look lonely and meager. Well, it works just the opposite as well. Feed the eye and fool the stomach. Even though logic may tell the child his or her portion is not bigger, logic has very little to do with eating. If the portion looks to be larger than everyone else's, it will be larger.

3. *Dress up the plate.* If your kid has decided that he wants, let us say, a hamburger, don't serve him one lonely little hamburger and let it go at that. Dress up the plate with items calculated to make the portion look like a meal, not a punishment. Some salad will do nicely—even if he doesn't want it. A slice of raw onion, or cooked onion. A small dab of ketchup. A tablespoon of cottage cheese. Let the cheese overflow the plate. Nothing is more satisfactory than to see an overflowing plate; it immediately provokes one to think there is more food there than one can eat. Sound silly? Well—how clever is being overweight? You think the way your child has been eating before is smart?

4. *When you serve, don't serve from a central dish on the table.* All plates should be filled in the kitchen. Not only does this prevent the immediate availablilty of "seconds" but it takes away even the notion that there is more food than is on the plate. As mentioned earlier, it is best to cook only the amount that you think can be eaten at the sitting; however, in many instances this is not possible. So cover your bets by keeping the central dish under cover—and, if seconds are asked for, as far as you are concerned there are none available.

5. *Package and freeze any leftovers in individual portions.* Again, this prevents, or at least makes more difficult, the "looting" of food that is all too likely to happen when leftovers are around.

Each dish, if possible, should be marked as to whom it is for for the following day, so that if its contents are interfered with, this will readily show. Of course we are overemphasizing the matter—but remember, we are dealing with a child, and in the case of continually bringing to a child's attention changes of habit pattern, overemphasis is a necessity. There is nothing subtle about being fat. You must fight fire with fire, and leave subtlety to the thin kids. Fat kids, in my experience, want to have a certain amount of fuss made over them, provided the fuss doesn't degenerate into "nagging."

6. *Turn out the refrigerator light.* I have known parents to remove it entirely. This does make rummaging in the frig more of a hassle than a pleasure, and while the ploy can be overcome, it may just make the endeavor more trouble than it is worth. I have had parents tell me that "my child is on his honor not to eat after dinner. When I take out the refrigerator light, aren't I telling him I don't trust him?" Of course you are. Honor has nothing to do with eating. The fat child is no less honorable than the thin one. To put any child on their honor as far as food is concerned is to give to eating a sense of exaltation that only makes it more important. It also makes the child feel more guilty when he or she goes off the diet. And, guilt is a good provoker of feeding.

No, I don't approve of mixing honor and food. The rules should be laid down at the beginning. The child that is fat is sick. He or she is sick because he or she is a food addict. While there is no shame in this, it is not an illness the child can conquer by him- or herself. That is why the parents are going to work with him or her. Taking the bulb out of the refrigerator, as well as all the other hints I have mentioned, is part of the way in which stumbling blocks are put in the child's way to help change behavior. Honor simply has nothing to do with the case.

FOR KIDS

Drink a large glass of water before each meal. This serves several functions. For one thing, it keeps the body hydrated and maintains a positive water balance. For another, it fills the stomach, getting rid of many of the "pangs" associated with hunger. Cold water will actually cut down on some of the peristaltic action of the intestines associated with the hunger syndrome. This activity also gives you a chance to sit back and decide just how hungry you are. If you think water is too bland a drink, you can jazz it up a bit with lemon or lime juice—and, for variety, you can substitute *salt-free seltzer* or Perrier water. The more water you drink during the day—eight eight-ounce glasses is a good figure if you can get that much down—the better off you will be. Water is a lot healthier drink than soda and even than diet soda. If you develop a good water-drinking habit, emphasized before meals, you will have taken a large step on the road to permanent weight loss.

Slow down your eating. The fact is that many kids, fat or thin, eat rather like sharks. The faster the mouth moves, the poorer the digestive processs, the less apt will you be to satisfy hunger. If you will learn to chew each mouthful of food till it is liquid, you will be satiating your mouth and will, therefore, be eating less. Gobblers eat more than selective chewers. Since it is debatable how much chewing makes a substance liquid in the mouth, I suggest that each mouthful be chewed ten to twelve times—no less—and that, at least at the beginning, you should count chews. This can be a tedious way to eat, but there is really no other way to provoke the habit. Once learned, it takes only the smallest amount of daily self-supervision to keep the activity on tap.

Make the meal last at least twenty-five minutes. It's amazing how fast many people eat—kids eat fastest of all. Going right along with the second point above, chewing each bite at least ten to twelve times, is taking longer at the meal itself. Obviously the meal will be automatically extended if longer chewing is activated, but there are other ways to extend the meal. The best way is to pause between bites—come up for air, as it were. You are not an eating machine, and you are not going to get a prize for the rapidity with which you pack your meal away. I assume you have been looking forward to eating, that eating is fun, that part of the fun is tasting the food, but a lot of the fun comes from enjoying the sight and smell of it as well. The meal should be a social occasion as well as a "fill the stomach" occasion. One boy recently remarked to me that it was almost time for him to "garbage up." He was referring to his own particular eating pattern. Having heard about his eating habits from his mother, I told him I could describe it no more effectively.

After sitting down to a meal, count to ten before actually starting to eat. Once again, this is a slowing-down process, an amount of time allowed to catch your breath and think rather than plunging mindlessly into the food. One habit that seems to be going by the board—literally—in many households is the saying of Grace before meals. This endeavor, religious motivations aside, tended to help prepare the digestive processes by giving them time. It aided good eating habits by preventing the taking of the food for granted, by covering it with an aura of respect. If you don't respect food, it won't respect you. "The pause that refreshes," though a slogan invented for a particular soft drink, can be turned to good account when used to describe the beginning of a meal. Remember, the faster you eat, the more you eat. So take your time.

Only eat when sitting down at a table with food on the plate. This means no snacks in other rooms, no wandering around the house with food in your mouth or on your plate. Have a specific room calculated as the "eating" room. It is then easy to catch yourself when you begin to nibble elsewhere. Part of this idea is to stop the eating in bed or eating in the bedroom that many kids get into the habit of doing. What this does is associate bedroom studytime, TV time, with eating. If eating becomes associated with any room in the house other than a specific one for the purpose, any activity done in such a room will automatically begin to call forth thoughts of food.

When you eat, that's all you do. This is important. There should be no other activity going on at the time. If there is, the eating activity will become secondary to what is happening. TV should be turned off during the eating process. If you are busy watching TV, you are really eating as a background to this particular stimulus. Certainly you are paying only minimal attention to your food. You begin eating like a machine, almost subconsciously, while your conscious attention is focused on the TV—or engaged in any other activity, such as reading, doing homework, having an argument with parents or brothers and sisters. It has been proved that the best way for kids—or, for that matter, grown-ups—to eat is to concentrate on the meal in hand and not have this concentration diluted by any other activity. Eating is enjoyable, after all. Why spoil it by not concentrating?

Slow down the eating pattern by putting knife and fork down between bites. In this manner, you are able to make sure you are chewing properly and that you are not gorging your mouth with food.

Don't let anyone con you into eating when you're not hungry. Three meals a day are not necessary, and I do not feel it is desirable for everyone—children as well as adults—to have to eat three times a day. Nor will it be necessary, when using the menu plan that will be shown in the next chapter, for all the food provided to be eaten just because it is listed.

IN GENERAL

There are factors based on individual habits that lead many children to overeat that simply can't be specified because they are too variable. Both parents and kids should try to ferret these out and, once discovered, change them. In addition, there may be physiological reasons for obesity. With adolescent girls the menstrual period may play a large part in weight gain. The best way I have found to encourage these youngsters is to assure them that the scale doesn't measure fat. It measures weight. They can be heavier without being fatter. Adolescent girls in their premenstrual phase can become mightily depressed. Such depression, added to by the frustration of weight gain, can end up driving them to eat more, not less. Patience and soothing words can do much at this point. If these kids don't get the support they especially need at this time from their parents, they will look for it in the refrigerator.

In the long run, kids must understand that it is not all that difficult to lose weight. It is, in fact, much too easy. That is why so many take off weight only to put it back on—because looking back it seemed not so difficult after all. Hopefully, this will not happen to them on this plan. It surely will not if they go on the maintenance portion. But there is no reason for them to think they will not be able to lose. All they have to do is try. Trying means success. The failures are sitting back eating, not trying.

EXERCISE

Proper control of one's weight—kid or adult—calls for energy expenditure in the form of exercise. Many people make the assumption that all children just naturally exercise as part of their daily routine. In fact, they do not. I am not going to go into all of the reasons to persuade kids why exercise is good for them. Probably you, as parents, have already told them—from your prone position on the sofa. But here's a table that may point up the idea, since it gives rather a graphic demonstration of the way any activity burns off calories (read, fat!):

CALORIES SPENT EACH
MINUTE FOR VARIOUS
ACTIVITIES

Activity	Calories per minute
Resting in bed	1.2
Sitting (normal)	1.4
Sitting (reading)	1.4
Sitting (eating)	1.6
Sitting (playing cards)	1.7
Standing (normal)	1.6
Standing (light activity)	2.8
Kneeling	1.4
Squatting	2.2
Football	10.1
Basketball	8.6
Ping-Pong	4.8
Bowling	8.1
Swimming	12.1
Golf	5.5

Activity	Calories per minute
Tennis	7.0
Walking (indoors)	3.4
Walking (outdoors)	6.1
Walking (downstairs)	7.6
Walking (upstairs)	20.0
Showering	3.7
Dressing	3.7
Making beds	5.3
Washing clothes	2.9
Mopping floors	5.3
Badminton	2.8
Rowing	8.0
Sailing	2.6
Playing pool	3.0
Dancing	4.0
Horseback riding	3.0

I have tried to cover most activities in which kids indulge. Try to get the kids to pick a few of the activities they enjoy, to get involved, and watch the weight come off. Keep in mind that you don't have to plunge right into the most violent forms of exercise, either as a kid or adult. It is much more healthy to make a moderate increase in daily activity day by day. Too many individuals limit their exercising to spurts of activity on the weekend. Remember, also, that the length of time you exercise is more important than how strenuous the exercise is. Getting the entire body involved is much more helpful than flexing a couple of sets of muscles. A one-mile walk will use up approximately a hundred calories compared to ten calories that you use up in twenty minutes of strenuous arm exercises. It may be more convenient to use the exerciser than to take the walk—but, as I have been pointing out, convenience is one of the ways your child got fat.

8

A Cycle of Successful Menu Plans

THE PICTURE

Before the child starts the actual plan, a picture should be taken. You can use Polaroid or a regular camera, color or black and white, but the picture should be taken as follows: two views of the body from head to knees, both full face and from the side. These two pictures establish peremptorily what the problem really looks like; we don't want to play guessing games. Toward this end, I find it is best that when taking the pictures the child wear fairly tight-fitting clothing; certainly getting the child a larger suit or dungarees prior to taking the picture, as one parent recently did, so "he will look better" is directly opposed to what the picture taking is all about. Show the child the pictures; keep the photographs. Then, as the child progresses in his weight loss, say at every fifteen pounds or so, take the same two views again. It is amazing how different the pictures will begin to look, even though the child may actually *feel* very little in the way of difference. By actually showing him—"Look, there is a difference, you can see it in the pictures"—you keep his attention engaged and his desire to lose weight constantly fueled.

MEASUREMENTS

All my patients have a specific measurement chart, as shown below:

	Measure Nude Tonight and Weekly						Goal	
Date								
Weight								
Chest ⊙ ⊙								
Waist ⊙								
Hips ( )								
Thighs ½								
Date								
Weight								
Chest								
Waist								
Hips								
Thighs								

Symbols represent the following: chest—nipples; waist—belly button; hips—the widest part; thighs—halfway between knee and groin (1 thigh).

Measurements are taken weekly and are written directly onto the chart. And while there is a place on the chart for the weight as well, it is critical to make sure that the child doesn't begin living on the scale. Normal body weight varies from day to day and within each day. The scale should not be a measure of punishment or reward. It should be only a guide.

It is interesting to keep in mind that weight loss and loss in inches do not always correspond. Often they decide to be contrary. A child, especially since he is growing, can lose inches far more readily than actual pounds. He or she should not be disappointed when this occurs, but, on the contrary, be proud of the fact. I have had children, in the course of a week, lose no weight at all on one of the pre-dieting cycles, yet lose a lot of inches. In general, a good inch loss one week can be said to prefigure a good loss of weight the next week, but this is not always true, so it should not be depended upon as a crutch to prop up falling confidence. All the same, it may well happen that way. The important thing is that the child take note of his or her inches so that all guesswork is proscribed. Measurements should *not* be taken at any areas not noted on the chart, or this, like constant weighing, will soon begin to drive everyone crazy. Let the child take his or her own measurements if he or she wishes; if not, the same parent should do it each time so that the amount of pull on the tape measure is approximately the same. I have picked areas to measure that are easy to find again: the chest at the nipple line, the waist at the belly button, the hips at the widest part (where the joint can be felt to move), and the thighs approximately halfway between knee and groin. A fairly simple way to go back to the same spot here is to make a span of the hand stretching from the little finger on the knee to where the thumb falls. This will provide an accurate enough and rapid guide.

Once the pictures have been taken and studied and the measurement card is understood, cyclic dieting is ready to begin. The only other tool that may be necessary is a food diary. This is merely a piece of paper, divided into the days of the week, that will be used to keep track of what is actually eaten and drunk. I employ food diaries rather as a check on the basic plan than a constant routine, since so many children find it rather a drag to keep writing things down.

BASIC MENU PLANS (1200–1500 CALORIES) FOR SUCCESSFUL ADOLESCENTS

As I said at the beginning, I cannot treat each child as an individual since I do not know him or her. I can deal in generalities, and you, the parent, together with your overweight adolescent, guided by the advice of your doctor, must pick out the details. The menus here will provide approximately 1,200 to 1,500 calories per day. You may want to take in fewer than this amount. If so, and if this is agreeable, you might try this for a day or so by diminishing the items as given. Remember, your stomach doesn't know the time of day, nor does it care. Only the food industry cares. Look what they've cared to do to you.

Remember the rules of eating. Not all the food in any individual meal must be eaten at that time. It may be carried over to the next meal. The sequence of meals is not important, nor is it necessary to eat all the meals in the course of the day. It depends on your child. Any of the days can be repeated. I have made this plan very simple to follow. If your son or daughter is at school during the lunch meal, he or she must bring lunch from home. *No substitutions please;* all vegetables either steamed or stir-fried.

DAY 1

(As every day, eight 8-ounce glasses of water throughout the day)

BREAKFAST
4 ounces orange juice
2 eggs, boiled or poached
1 piece Ry-Krisp or similar 25-calorie bread
8 ounces skim milk

LUNCH
⅔ cup cottage cheese
Salad (sliced tomato, lettuce, and cucumbers; 2 cups total) with 2 tablespoons oil and vinegar dressing
½ cup unsweetened fruit cocktail
1 can diet soda

DINNER
6 ounces broiled liver
½ cup cooked peas, steamed or stir-fried
1 cup cooked carrots, steamed or stir-fried
1 cup cabbage salad (grated cabbage with vinegar)
Tea, coffee, or 1 can diet soda

*BEDTIME **   1 raw apple

Day 2

BREAKFAST   ½ grapefruit
                              ½ cup low-fat cottage cheese
                              1 piece Melba toast
                              8 ounces skim milk

LUNCH   4 ounces boiled shrimp
                              1 hard-boiled egg
                              Salad (lettuce, celery, green
                                  pepper, radishes, onions; 6
                                  ounces total) with 2 tablespoons
                                  oil and vinegar dressing
                              1 piece whole-wheat toast
                              ½ cup pineapple (unsweetened
                                  canned or fresh)
                              1 can diet soda

DINNER   6 ounces broiled fillet of sole
                              ½ cup baked potato
                              1 cup cooked beets
                              Salad (3 lettuce leaves, 2 slices
                                  tomato)
                              1 tangerine
                              8 ounces skim milk

BEDTIME   1 cup plain yogurt

Day 3

BREAKFAST   1 orange
                              ⅔ cup cold cereal (nonsweet
                                  cereal)
                              1 egg, boiled or poached
                              8 ounces skim milk (may use part
                                  for cereal)

*You may, if you wish, use your bedtime snacks at school for
an afternoon "break." This is variable.

LUNCH	4 ounces canned salmon 1 slice whole-wheat bread Salad (lettuce, celery, tomato, green pepper; 6 ounces total) with 1 teaspoon diet mayonnaise 1 raw apple
DINNER	6 ounces roast beef ½ cup mushrooms (raw, fried in nonstick pan, or canned) ½ cup cooked broccoli Mixed green salad (lettuce, cucumber, green peppers, celery; 8 ounces total) with 3 tablespoons oil and vinegar ½ cup unsweetened canned pears 1 can diet soda
BEDTIME	1 cup skim milk

Day 4

BREAKFAST	½ cup orange juice 2 eggs, boiled or poached 1 slice whole-wheat toast 1 cup skim milk
LUNCH	4 ounces canned salmon Salad (lettuce, tomato, watercress; 8 ounces total) with 1 tablespoon diet mayonnaise 1 piece whole-wheat toast ½ cup sliced pineapple (no juice if canned, preferably fresh) 1 cup skim milk
DINNER	½ cup tomato juice 8 ounces roast veal

½ cup baked potato
½ cup cooked string beans
½ cup cooked beets
1 raw apple
1 can diet soda

BEDTIME

1 raw apple
1 cup skim milk

Day 5

BREAKFAST

½ grapefruit
1 egg, boiled or poached
2 thin slices whole-wheat toast
1 cup skim milk

LUNCH

⅔ cup cottage cheese
Fruit salad (½ cup orange
    segments, ½ cup diced fresh
    pear, 4 ounces escarole)
1 thin slice whole-wheat toast with
    1 teaspoon butter or margarine
    or ½ teaspoon diet jelly
1 can diet soda

DINNER

1 cup tomato juice
8 ounces roast beef
6 ounces eggplant (sliced and fried
    in nonstick pan)
½ cup cooked beets
Salad (celery, cucumber, green
    pepper, mushrooms, onions)
    with either plain lemon dressing
    or 2 tablespoons oil and vinegar
    dressing
1 piece melba toast
1 raw apple
Tea, 1 can diet soda

BEDTIME

1 cup plain yogurt

DAY 6

BREAKFAST

1 orange
1 egg, boiled or poached
2 strips well-done bacon
1 piece melba toast
1 cup skim milk

LUNCH

Chicken salad (4 ounces cooked chicken breast, 6 ounces lettuce, tomato, celery, onion) with ¼ cup oil and vinegar dressing
1 tangerine
1 can diet soda

DINNER

8 ounces broiled flounder
½ cup baked potato
1 cup cooked brussels sprouts
½ cup cooked winter squash
½ cup fruit cocktail
1 cup skim milk

DAY 7

BREAKFAST

1 orange
⅔ cup cornflakes
1 cup skim milk (may use part for cereal)
Tea or coffee

LUNCH

½ cup unsweetened grapefruit juice
1 slice whole-wheat bread
4 ounces cooked crabmeat
Salad (½ cup celery, ½ cup lettuce, ½ cup tomato) with 2 tablespoons oil and vinegar dressing
1 can diet soda, tea or coffee

DINNER

6 ounces breast of chicken, broiled
1 slice whole-wheat bread
Salad (½ cup cooked cauliflower,
    ½ cup lettuce, ½ cup escarole)
    with 1 tablespoon diet
    mayonnaise
1 cup cooked beets
1 cup skim milk

BEDTIME

1 raw apple or a small ball of
    cottage cheese with a dash of
    vanilla and nutmeg

SPEED SUBSTITUTES—INCREASING THE WEIGHT LOSS

Adolescents are growing people, and it is critical, as I have repeatedly mentioned throughout this book, that health comes first. To make certain that your child is getting the requisite vitamins and minerals he needs, he should take, unfailingly, a good vitamin/mineral supplement each day. It is also a good idea to stay in touch with your family doctor and report to him any particular problems that may occur. This does not mean that your child will not feel well on this plan. On the contrary, it is likely he or she will have never felt better. However, individual variation being what it is, and the power of the mind as it surveys the "bleak" prospects of going on a diet, may provide the dieter with occasional feelings of discomfort. These should be checked out, or at least reported, before going on with any diet.

More to the point is that your child, the previously "impossibly overweight" kid, will suddenly find he doesn't even need all the food that is provided on a daily basis. If this is the case, you may want to substitute some of the "Food Blocks" listed below in place of any one of those given in the cycle. I call these "speed substitutes," since they help to get the weight off a little faster. Speed substitutes should not be used if the child is more hungry with them. In this case, continue with the basic cycle as written, or form your own from the diet pattern at the end of the chapter. You don't have to choose a substitute every day, and even if you end up not choosing any of them, it's still nice to know they are there. Watch the salt—use a minimum amount—a salt substitute is best if tolerated.

SS FOOD BLOCK 1
½ orange
1 hard-boiled egg
1 cup skim milk

SS FOOD BLOCK 2
1 cup clear beef broth
1 four-ounce hamburger
1 tablespoon cottage cheese
1 cup skim milk

SS FOOD BLOCK 3
3 medium boiled shrimp with 1 teaspoon cocktail sauce
1 piece Ry-Krisp
1 tablespoon cottage cheese

SS FOOD BLOCK 4
1 slice whole-wheat toast with 1 teaspoon diet jelly
½ cup orange juice
1 cup whole milk

SS FOOD BLOCK 5
1 cup beef bouillon
2 broiled all-beef frankfurters (no rolls, please) with 1 tablespoon mustard
1 cup skim milk

SS FOOD BLOCK 6
1 egg, fried or scrambled in nonstick pan
1 piece Ry-Krisp
1 cup skim milk

SS FOOD BLOCK 7
1 cup vegetable soup
4 ounces water-pack tuna
1 can diet soda

SS FOOD BLOCK 8
6 ounces fillet of sole or similar nonoily fish

2 pieces Ry-Krisp
½ cup cooked broccoli
1 cup whole milk

SS FOOD BLOCK 9

1 egg, sunny side up, fried in
     nonstick pan
1 piece Ry-Krisp
1 cup skim milk

SS FOOD BLOCK 10

1 cup clam chowder
4 ounces boiled shrimp
½ cup boiled or baked potato
1 can diet soda

SS FOOD BLOCK 11

4 ounces steak or 6 ounces lamb
     or veal, broiled or fried in
     nonstick pan
½ cup cooked broccoli
1 tossed green salad (4 ounces
     total) with 1 tablespoon oil and
     vinegar dressing
1 cup skim milk

SS FOOD BLOCK 12

4 ounces orange juice
½ cup cornflakes
1 cup whole milk

SS FOOD BLOCK 13

1 cup low-calorie bouillon, broth,
     or consommé
Salad (1 sliced hard-boiled egg,
     several lettuce leaves, 2 slices
     tomato, 1 sliced carrot, 2 slices
     green pepper; no dressing)
1 can diet soda

SS FOOD BLOCK 14

½ cup unsweetened fruit cocktail
3 ounces broiled steak
1 medium broiled tomato
½ cup cooked broccoli
1 cup skim milk

SS FOOD BLOCK 15	¼ cantaloupe 1 hard-boiled egg 1 cup whole milk
SS FOOD BLOCK 16	1 cup beef bouillon 1 four-ounce hamburger 1 can diet soda
SS FOOD BLOCK 17	1 cup tomato juice 4 ounces sliced white meat of chicken or turkey 3 medium asparagus spears 1 cup whole milk
SS FOOD BLOCK 18	½ grapefruit 1 cup whole milk

SS FOOD BLOCK 19	Salad (4 lettuce leaves, 1 medium
	  sliced tomato, 2 slices green
	  pepper, 1 slice onion, ½ medium
	  sliced carrot, 3 slices cucumber)
	  with 2 tablespoons oil and
	  vinegar dressing, pepper

SS FOOD BLOCK 20	1 cup beef bouillon 3 ounces roast beef 1 piece Ry-Krisp 1 cup whole milk

The above can be substituted for any of the meals on the basic plan provided your child is:

1. Drinking eight eight-ounce glasses of water daily.
2. Taking daily multivitamin-mineral tablets.
3. Maintaining a good weight loss.
4. Feeling well.
5. Feeling he doesn't need all the food that is supplied on the basic plan. I do not suggest that you substitute more than one food block per day.

BONUS FOODS—THE CALORIE PICKUP SPECIAL

If your child's weight loss has been very good, or if he's feeling a bit bored, you might like to try one of these bonus treats. Use them only as special events, not as routine, "I've got it coming to me, I've been so good today" incidentals. They can all be whipped up in a blender or shaken in a covered jar.

Tomato Surprise
(60 calories)

Combine ½ cup buttermilk, ½ cup tomato juice, a pinch of salt substitute, drop of Worcestershire sauce in a jar with a lid or a blender; shake or blend until smooth. This will make your child sit up and take notice; it will also fill him or her up.

The Yo-Ho Shake
(100 calories)

Combine ½ cup plain yogurt, ¾ cup unsweetened orange juice, a dash of vanilla in a jar or blender and shake or blend until smooth. Smooth and tangy.

The Up Beet
(80 calories)

Blend together ½ cup plain yogurt, ⅔ cup beet juice, a touch of black pepper and dill. It's a dilly.

The No-Sour Grape Shape
(70 calories)

Blend together ½ cup skim milk, a dash of vanilla, 1 tablespoon unsweetened grape juice (or even 1½ tablespoons), an egg white, and a dash of cinnamon. Make it nice and tart with a little lemon juice.

THE RED ROVER
(60 calories)

Blend ½ cup plain yogurt, 1 cup tomato juice, and salt substitute and pepper to taste.

THE EAST FEAST
(80 calories)

Combine ½ cup orange juice, ½ cup unsweetened grape juice, and 4 ounces skim milk in a jar with a lid. Shake well. When the mixture froths up, add some shreds of coconut or shredded pineapple.

THE BUTTER-APPLE SPECIAL
(90 calories)

Blend together ½ cup unsweetened applesauce and ½ cup buttermilk. A nice, thick drink.

THE ORANGE PEEL DEAL
(90 calories)

Blend ½ cup skim milk, ½ cup unsweetened orange juice, 1 stiffly beaten egg white, ½ cup carbonated water, and 1 teaspoon grated orange peel.

THE COFFEE BREAK
(70 calories)

Combine in a glass 1 cup skim milk, 1 teaspoon instant coffee, ½ cup carbonated water, and several dashes of vanilla or almond extract. Pour the mix from one glass to another; it foams up and will fill him or her up as well.

VEGETARIAN'S DELIGHT
(80 calories)

1 cup buttermilk mixed with 1 tablespoon shredded cucumber, ¼ teaspoon finely grated onion, 2 teaspoons finely grated celery, 1 tablespoon shredded carrot, ½ teaspoon lemon juice. Everything but the kitchen sink—but how nice it is.

If you have a blender and some imagination, you can mix up all sorts of interesting combinations, some of which may take your kid's breath away, many of which will help take his weight away. It's a question of taste, time, and preference. Choose combinations that he finds appealing and give them a try. A good base is powdered skim milk, protein in a very flexible form. There is almost nothing in the way of protein-vitamin pickups with which it doesn't combine. Give it a try. It always amazes me how quick people are to rush out and spend money on the latest commercial preparation that, for one reason or another (usually clever advertising), has become a fad. Urge your child to whip up his own combinations, using as starter samples those I've provided. The use of the skim-milk base together with fresh fruits and vegetables will provide him or her with unending combinations. Encouraging and helping your child to come up with a delicious and low-calorie treat will help him in the battle to lose weight.

To see how easy it is to please adolescent palates with new and nutritious drinks, take a glance at some of the drinks listed below, which can readily take the place of those omnipresent sugar-laden sodas.

A FEW INTERESTING DRINK MIXES

1. Unsweetened cranberry juice combined with an ounce or two of diet 7-Up makes a treat for the palate that your kid never got at the corner soda market. It's a lot better for him than Coke—and a lot easier on your pocketbook.

2. Mixing different types of juices together to make a new combination is always fun. The commercial drinks are already moving in that direction. Tomato juice is a good base; two variations are equal parts of tomato juice and celery juice or tomato juice and carrot juice. For a little extra zing you can add some seltzer, which is calorie-free!

3.   Seltzer is also good with orange juice. This serves a double purpose in diluting the juice (O.J. is fairly high in the calorie department) as well as giving the drink a bit of a kick. Since I grow a lot of fresh mint, I use it wherever possible in drinks, and one use is here. Chop up the leaf rather fine and sprinkle it in.

4.   Tea, of course, is always good as a starter. All sorts of teas are available in the stores. Start your child on the tea habit. Herb teas, because of their delicate taste, are nice to mix with other items to help bring out their flavor, and they don't contain tannin or caffeine. A small amount of orange or lemon juice with sprinkles of powdered ginger or cinnamon (use spices as much as possible—they contain no calories but add a great deal of flavor) will make a delicious drink either hot or iced.

The above are, of course, only random selections, but they should give you the idea. You want to present your chubby child with a whole new adventure; he or she has heard the old routine too many times by now to be terribly impressed by it. And you really must impress your child—and keep him or her impressed—if you want to keep his or her attention on losing weight. As I keep saying, the best way is for you to join in.

SPENDING THE ADOLESCENT'S CALORIE BUDGET

Depending, of course, on how much your child has to lose, his intake must be budgeted to a certain extent. There are some general regulations here; keeping these in mind will allow you, the parent, to develop menus other than those laid down in these pages, to continue over a period of weeks or months the weight loss established with the aid of these plans. Foods should be selected from the following list, on a daily basis, to the calculated amounts:

Skimmed milk	About 2 cups
Whole milk	About 2 cups
Cottage cheese (low fat)	About 1 cup to 1½ cups
Eggs	1 per day, at most 9 a week (The method of preparing eggs is essential, since the 75-calorie value generally assigned to eggs only applies to the boiled egg or the egg fried in a nonstick pan. You can add a lot of calories to a food, like eggs, in the way you prepare it.)
Selected meat, fish, or poultry	1 medium portion per day (I prefer to emphasize fish and fowl rather than the red meat so many families think it essential to eat every day. Again, the way you prepare the foods makes a big difference in the calorie budgeting.)
Vegetables and fruits	At least 2 cups of any of the following should be provided per day: asparagus, bean sprouts, beans (string), beet greens, broccoli, cabbage, cauliflower, celery, chard, collards, cucumber, dandelion greens, endive, escarole, kale, lettuce, mushrooms, mustard greens, parsley, peppers, pimientos, poke greens, radishes, rhubarb, sauerkraut, spinach, squash, turnip greens, watercress, all fruits, tomatoes, and tomato juice

Grains	Wheat bread, 2 thin slices twice a day, grain cereal 3 to 4 times a week
Water	8 eight-ounce glasses a day as soon as possible (this may have to be worked up to)
Salt	As little as possible from the salt shaker

I like to keep the adolescent's calorie total at approximately 1,600. Naturally this varies, depending on my assessment of the patient. You, the parent, guided by the child's doctor, must make your own assessment of the situation and act according to the guidelines I have furnished.

PREPARING THE FOOD SO YOUR KID WILL LOVE IT BUT IT WON'T HATE HIM

The food on these menus can be prepared in many ways: you can broil, fry, barbecue, bake it. It can be eaten raw if that's the choice. Deep-fat frying is restricted; so is breading. It is important that you do not allow your child to become bored with what you are presenting him or her. One way to prevent this is to use a great variety of seasonings. Employ them moderately. Some seasonings are salty, such as onion salt and garlic salt, and should be used in moderation. Instead use garlic and onion powder, which are salt free. Don't overuse saccharin, since for many kids taking anything faintly resembling sugar just gives them an automatic itch for candy. We want to diminish, not enhance, the sugar desire. In this regard let me say a word about honey. It is surprising to me how many people consider honey an innocuous substance just because it is "natural" sugar. Cane sugar, sucrose, is also a "natural" sugar; the same sugar is in honey—and it is as disastrous to the overweight body as the refined sugar on the table.

Keeping these few things in mind, it is certainly possible to create tasty dishes that will keep the fat adolescent intrigued and comfortable. He or she must understand that you are helping without becoming a guard. Keep the refrigerator stocked with fruits and vegetables that are on the plan for snacking; remember, if it isn't in the house, he or she isn't going to eat it— at least at home.

9

A Teenager's Guide to Dieting (Mostly Girls)

Once again I'd like to direct my remarks to the "fat kid" himself or, even more specifically, herself. At this stage of your life, day-to-day existence is complicated enough without more weight on your shoulders—your *own* weight. Nevertheless, it is there. How can you get out from under? Are you doomed to be fat forever? Should you just try to make the best of the situation or can you really do something about it?

First of all, let us keep in mind the fact that not all weight gain—even that of an overweight person such as you—is fat. Remember that your body is still growing, and occasionally this growth precedes an actual increase in height by first laying down an increase in body fat. So don't get discouraged so fast. Try to take everything, every possibility, into account. This is especially true when you are on a diet and appear to be putting on weight regardless of how "good" you have been. And remember that for boys and girls there *is* a difference, one that is almost enough during this time to divide them into separate species. Boys have a tendency to grow in bulk, what is called "body mass," even more rapidly than they grow in height. The sexual differences that have been lurking behind the scenes through childhood are now, at this point, going to break forth almost explosively. Needless to say, this complicates every-thing—even your emotions about being fat.

Especially in girls, these adolescent/teenage sexual changes can make for a weight problem even where none may have existed before. It is not unusual for me to find a new patient in my office, brought in by a troubled parent, who says to me in an incredulous voice, "Doctor, I've never been fat in my life; now look at me. And it seems to be just beginning."

Many doctors will regard such a young lady with the suspicion that she has all along been a heavy eater, fill her full of guilt feelings, and literally drive her to food in frustration.

What most girls don't know about themselves and their body weight could fill a book. I don't intend to fill this one with all those dry statistics, but a few items along this line should be of interest. For one thing, just before entering adolescence, at about age eleven or twelve, most girls experience a sudden spurt of growth (not fat) that is the prelude to becoming a woman. About this point the menstrual period starts. Also, fat deposits begin to fill in those graceful curves, providing waists, busts, and thighs in proportion to bodily demands. All well and good—but at the same time that this rise in fat tissue begins (and it normally continues in girls till late adolescence, say age eighteen) there occurs somewhat of a drop in growth. To her horror, the young lady begins to feel and look stocky. It is precisely at this time she should take care and start cutting down on the number of calories she is taking in, watching her weight carefully. If she continues eating as she has been, she is likely to find alarming amounts of weight coming on. Then the problem can be compounded in that, feeling fat, she begins to stay more by herself, avoiding the exercise groups, the plain physical activity that can help her burn off the excess fat. Adolescence is at best such a mixed-up time that if a girl begins to sulk about by herself, she is very likely to begin to use food as a consolation process—just the element she certainly doesn't need.

Boys don't have the same problem as girls. As they get further and further into adolescence, this initial deposit of fat suddenly burns itself up in growth. That is not to say that adolescence isn't as disturbing a time for boys as for girls, but girls do have more of a problem achieving a weight balance.

THE MENSTRUAL CYCLE

Many teenagers, especially at the beginning of this time span, have irregular periods. Whether regular or irregular, it is likely that when your period comes you will weigh more. You will feel bloated, probably, and can certainly make the connection between the fluid you are retaining and the weight gain. Even if you don't feel bloated, you should be able, logically, to connect the one physiologic event with the realities of the scale. However, teenagers, like their overweight adult counterparts, are not always logical—and certainly not where weight is concerned. In fact, logic is a poor weapon in this regard, because emotion seems to be the controlling factor.

"My heavens," one seventeen-year-old girl said as she stepped on my office scale. "I've gained three pounds. And I was so good." And she started to cry.

I pointed out to her that, according to my records, she was premenstrual. She admitted it, abating not a jot of her tears, and said, "I know. It's such a depressing time for me anyway. And now I'm even more depressed."

That's what I mean by allowing emotion to rule your reason. Sure, we all do it more often, perhaps, than we even realize. But where weight is concerned, it can be a deadly process—and one that should be reversed.

"I feel like going home now and eating all the things I've denied myself," my patient then said. "After all, what's the use?"

"But," I said, "if you do that, you'll gain fat."

"What difference does it make? I'm fat now."

"No," I said. "You've gained weight with your period, but that is not the same thing as gaining fat. The weight that you've put on will vanish with your period—sometimes when it starts, more often when it ends—but if you now go and add fat, that will remain after your period goes. Then you can use this real weight gain as an excuse that your diet doesn't work. I won't let you think that. I can't stop you from going home and bingeing, but I refuse to allow you to use your period as a copout." And that's the best advice I can give you, too.

A SPECIAL PROBLEM: THE PREGNANT TEENAGER

I mention this situation here because I have had pregnant teenagers brought to my office by parents anxious that their daughter lose weight in order to have an easier delivery. I think that few choices for her future can be more open to question. In instances where the pregnant teenager is already obese before pregnancy, getting pregnant certainly compounds her dietary problems, but trying to unravel them at this stage can make her general health worse, not better. For one thing, dietary surveys of pregnant teenagers have found inadequate protein and caloric intake even where the mother-to-be was not obese prior to pregnancy. Low intakes of iron, calcium, and vitamin A are also common.

Actually, the pregnant teenager requires more in the way of proper nutrition than does the pregnant adult female, since she is still growing herself. An adequate weight gain for a pregnant teenager could range from twenty-seven to thirty-five pounds. What happens if it is more than that? Such instances have to be individually calculated, though it is safe to say that any teenager who is grossly obese and who adds pregnancy to her list is flirting with disaster. In such a case some means should be established to exercise control over what this young mother is eating—both for her own safety and for that of her child. Teenage mothers already have a tendency to have smaller babies than more mature women. These smaller infants are more sensitive to the consequences of a difficult labor and can experience more complications during the first days of life than larger infants.

So there is no rule of thumb as far as getting overweight pregnant teenagers to lose weight. Such young people are not only physically on the edge, but generally mentally as well. Each must be treated as a specialized instance under the guidance of the family doctor, who should not attempt to guide their progress by any generalized plan, including this one. One thing, however, that can be assumed as a fairly standard treatment would be to provide all the supplements described in the preceding section. The pregnant teenager will almost certainly need plenty of them.

THE PILL

One of the special problems girls run into at this age is birth-control pills. There is no sense in trying to look the other way when this question comes up. Better to face the issue squarely. And the issue is that teenagers taking the Pill do need special attention as far as their weight is concerned. This is especially true if the girl is trying to lose weight at this time. Even on what is called a "reasonably balanced diet"—a most ambiguous phrase—girls can have problems weightwise with the Pill.

Some of the problems can be counteracted by knowing what is happening and taking appropriate steps, especially where the effects are less than obvious. One of the effects is: an increase of vitamin-A levels in the body. So you certainly would not want to be taking high doses of this vitamin while on contraceptive medications. I mention this particularly because, while routine supplementation with this vitamin is no problem, teenagers tend to suffer from skin difficulties, are horrified easily at such blemishes, and will dose themselves (at least in instances I am aware of) with many fad medications—one of which could be high doses of vitamin A. It is true that such doses are prescription items, but I suggest that before taking anything of this nature you tell your doctor you are on the Pill.

Calcium levels of the body also run higher when the Pill is being used, and since the Pill usually lessens the menstrual flow, the need for iron can be somewhat decreased. Many adolescents on iron pills for slight anemia can go off such supplements when on the Pill after suitable tests have determined this possibility.

There is a drop in the B-complex group, and it would be a good idea to cover this defect by making sure a good multivitamin is taken daily, as I constantly recommend throughout the book.

Perhaps more important to the mind of the girl on the Pill are the obvious physical changes it will cause in her—at least on a temporary basis. Almost inevitably I have found an initial weight gain. While some girls can start on the Pill without ever having this occur, I usually mention it as a very real probability. Much, if not all, of this initial gain is fluid retention due to the high levels of estrogen, one of the female hormones, now circulating in the body. You may feel bloated on the Pill. Indeed, you may go through a number of the signs of pregnancy: breasts can enlarge, nausea can occur—and, of course, a weight gain will be noted. It isn't necessary to have a fit of despair over all this, however. Such signs will eventually go away. The important thing is to get through them, after realizing what they come from. And, if you are lucky, you will not have any of them.

No matter how often I tell my female patients of these possibilities, they inevitably get dismayed when they don't lose weight during the initial stages of Pill-taking. I am used to this by now. You should get used to it to.

WHAT ABOUT WATER PILLS?

Speaking of the Pill reminds me that there are many other kinds of pills around, pills that are used for weight loss. Most popular are the diuretics, or "water pills," that many women, both adult and teenage, use to alleviate "bloating." This condition of feeling "stuffed with water," as one of my patients recently put it, seems to be a part of the female physiology—and has gotten into the female psyche as well. I would advise you not to consider water pills as the answer to losing weight. If your doctor has given them to you to help get you through your premenstrual swelling, much of which can be due to retained body fluid, that doesn't mean you should go on a steady diet of water pills. The tendency to think that "if a few are good, many are better" doesn't work out when it comes to these pills. I have had teenage girls come to my office who take two and three diuretics a day in the belief that if they do not, some sort of dam will burst inside them and they will be inundated by a mysterious flood of water. Believe me, that won't happen.

More important than water pills in keeping fluid retentive factors under control is salt intake. Teenagers tend to use a lot of salt, but even if they do not overuse the salt shaker (and from what I have observed in restaurants this is more the case than not), many of the so-called junk foods are rich in salt. Cut down on salt and in many instances you can throw your water pills away. In any event, you must get over the notion of thinking of your body as a giant sponge that must be squeezed out once in a while. The body water you get rid of by using constant and strong diuretics comes right back. In addition, the overuse of these pills can cause leg cramps (or more extreme reactions) through loss of potassium as well as injury to the kidneys. And, speaking of the difference between reason and emotion, it is certainly unreasonable to assume your body is too stupid to know what to do with its excess fluid. That is what you have kidneys for. It is true that diuretics, used judiciously, can be a comfort at times of hormone imbalance such as during or before the period. I would discourage their constant use in adults; certainly in teenagers it would be best, where possible, to do without them except in the very rare instance. Never think of them as "weight-loss" pills. The best diuretic I know, and the most natural and healthy one, is water. Drink—and you'll see the excess water drain out of you, you'll stay healthy, and you'll lose true weight as well, not just water weight. Interestingly (just to show the illogic of the whole proceeding) many teenagers on water pills take them with a full eight-ounce glass of orange juice to make up for potassium loss. The amount of unnecessary calories taken in with the juice more than makes up in weight gain—fat gain—for the temporary loss of water weight.

WHAT ABOUT VITAMINS AND MINERALS?

My feeling is that we are all overdosed on vitamins. As far as the average, healthy teen is concerned, unless a specific disorder exists, I cannot see why high doses of vitamins and minerals are necessary. I recommend taking one multivitamin with minerals daily. Yet I have seen numbers of both teens and adults who would feel quite insecure if they didn't take a full armamentarium of vitamins several times a day. Most of this is quite useless.

However, in one respect, the mineral iron, may be important, as far as girls are concerned. It is difficult for females of almost any age to maintain sufficient iron stores in their body. The menstrual period, of course, is a factor here. One way to replace and maintain iron stores is not by drinking wine, as is popularly supposed (even red wine does not build blood, store iron, or keep you any healthier in this regard than you would otherwise be), but by eating red meats, especially liver. But, if like most people you do not like liver, you may find that iron supplements will help. The teen may profit here by learning to eat iron-rich foods and thus avoid the pill route. However, I have found this kind of suggestion to my own patients pretty much a dead end.

One thing you should watch out for as far as many iron preparations are concerned is constipation. Since constipation is already a factor in many diets, it would not be a good idea to enhance the possibility of difficulty with it here. If you do go on iron, get a preparation that contains a stool softener. This will at least help to avoid a potential problem. You should also be aware that iron preparations tend to turn the stool dark. I have had several teenage patients who got scared to death at this, no one having warned them beforehand.

Iron should not be taken arbitrarily. Check with your physician. A simple blood test will show if you are iron deficient. If you are "borderline," you may find that going on iron will make all the difference as to how you feel. You want to feel your absolute best when engaged in a life-or-death struggle with your weight.

WHAT ABOUT ANOREXIA NERVOSA?

Since this is primarily a disease common to young girls, it is well to discuss it here. It can be a disaster. The disease is not entirely understood: it appears to be a total backlash against food. The girls I spoke to who had been through the process were intelligent overachievers—which doesn't mean that other types cannot get it. Whatever the triggering situation may be, the result is that the individual attempts to lose weight by maintaining strict control over her body—an attempt that can only be described as desperate. The goal is not only achieved but overdone—to such an extent that actual starvation begins to occur, accompanied by such dismaying symptoms as loss of hair and loss of the menstrual process. Eventually, if the disease is not arrested, death will occur. More and more of such cases keep coming to light.

As far as treatment is concerned, both medical and psychological care is necessary. This is not something the victim can treat on her own, nor can her parents help her. Hospitalization is recommended: first, because the individual must have the support of artificial methods to maintain health; second, to get the patient into an atmosphere totally removed from that in which the situation occurred.

Some of you girls reading this may have friends or acquaintances who were anorexics, and may thus be aware that the condition is completely curable. In fact, such individuals traveling this merry-go-round cycle can even become overweight—a situation that was not necessarily the case when they fell into anorexia. The problem is a strange one, but fortunately it is not widespread—though it is certainly more prevalent than many people realize. At the same time, the chance of your becoming anorexic is nonexistent if your attempt to lose weight is guided by a reasonable plan along medical lines. I mention the situation here not as a warning but rather as an example of the extremes into which people can fall where weight is the issue.

The following chart will give you an idea of some of the nutritional requirements for females. The caloric ranges are not meant to be representative of overweight or obese individuals. At the same time, when you calculate, as has been done, that the typical teenage menu (boys and girls combined) is about 4,100 calories per day, it can easily be seen that even the ratios of calories here would constitute a diet for most such individuals. Certainly such a high caloric intake would be disastrous for the more sedentary adults; for you, the teen, even handling it well for a while will almost certainly get you into trouble if you aren't already there.

Nutritional Requirements (Female)

	Ages 7–10 *	Ages 11–14	Ages 15–18	Ages 19–22	Ages 23–50
	66 lb. 54 in.	97 lb. 62 in.	119 lb. 65 in.	128 lb. 65 in.	128 lb. 65 in.
Calories **	2,400	2,400	2,100	2,100	2,000
Protein (g)	26	44	48	46	46
Vitamin A Activity (IU)	3,300	4,000	4,000	4,000	4,000
Vitamin D (IU)	400	400	400	400	400
Vitamin E Activity (IU)	10	10	11	12	12
Ascorbic Acid (mg)	40	45	45	45	45
Folacin (μg)	300	400	400	400	400
Niacin (mg)	16	16	14	14	13
Riboflavin (mg)	1.2	1.3	1.4	1.4	1.2
Thiamin (mg)	1.2	1.2	1.1	1.1	1.0

* Figures in this column also apply to males.
** Technically, the correct term here is "kilocalories" (1,000 calories = 1 calorie or 1 kilocalorie)

Source: National Research Council Recommended Daily Dietary Allowances, revised 1974. Food and Nutrition Board, National Academy of Sciences.

	Ages 7–10 *	Ages 11–14	Ages 15–18	Ages 19–22	Ages 23–50
	66 lb.	97 lb.	119 lb.	128 lb.	128 lb.
	54 in.	62 in.	65 in.	65 in.	65 in.
Vitamin B$_6$ (mg)	1.2	1.6	2.0	2.0	2.0
Vitamin B$_{12}$ (μg)	2.0	3.0	3.0	3.0	3.0
Calcium (mg)	800	1200	1200	800	800
Phosphorus (mg)	800	1200	1200	800	800
Iodine (μg)	110	115	115	100	100
Iron (mg)	10	18	18	18	18
Magnesium (mg)	250	300	300	300	300
Zinc (mg)	10	15	15	15	15

THE FAD DIET

It isn't only teenagers who are responsive to fads, of course; it's just that for some reason they seem to be most blamed for following them. Probably the worst kind of fad to follow is the fad diet.

Any reducing diet that provides only a temporary sort of relief from overweight is merely skirting the issue—and making a larger skirt for you directly after you go off the fad. Not only is this a disappointing comeuppance, but losing some weight—or even quite a bit of it—on some "magical" plan, then having the plan come to an end, gaining the weight again . . . and going through this process over and over makes it more and more difficult to keep losing in succeeding endeavors. No diet plan will work that does not teach you how to retrain basic eating habits. All of the factors that I have gone over in this book, plus others noted in one of my previous books, *Fat Free Forever*, must come into play for successful weight loss to be accomplished. By its very nature, weight loss must take place over a period of time. It can't occur immediately. To the anxious dieter—and teens have, in the main, too busy a life-style for absolute patience—any more, perhaps, than have the rest of us—it is easier to eat promises than facts. Unfortunately, it is these promises that eventually make you even fatter, more miserable than before. The best way to avoid this sort of situation is to *be reasonable* about your weight. And when the next fad diet comes down the pike—be it macrobiotic, Zen,vegetarian, Ox/ Yak Soup, or what have you, just step aside and let it pass. Don't hop on, because your disease—and overweight is a disease—won't hop on with you.

SUGAR AND YOUR PERIOD

Sugar used in moderation is not fattening. The problem, and one more prevalent among women, lies in its overuse, an insidious process almost similar to drug addiction. No one will get fat from a teaspoon of sugar in their tea. But three teaspoons in constant cups of tea will certainly provide an excess of calories that your body is likely unequipped to handle. The reason you may take several teaspoons rather than one is that, for many of us, one teaspoon is no longer enough for us to taste. Our taste buds have become blunted to sugar; we need more of it to enjoy the flavor. And this more becomes still more as we add to the three or four teaspoons the cakes and pies and ice creams that further feed our addiction—and in turn make us want more sugar. The drinking of sugared colas is a good example. Does one Coke really soothe your thirst? Or does it just soothe your sugar taste momentarily, providing, really, the itch for another?

The only way I myself have been able to live in an over-sugared world is to avoid the stuff altogether. That does not mean excluding all carbohydrates from the diet. You will find plenty of carbohydrates there. Yes, it is true that carbohydrates are broken down by the body to sugar. And, yes, it is true that the specific sugar, glucose, the only sugar that the body utilizes, is a specific energy requirement for the body—especially the brain. It is certainly necessary for the high-energy requirements of the adolescent, particularly the female, with her up and down hormone fluctuations. But that doesn't mean that refined table sugar is the answer. (Even brown sugar is certainly not the answer; I classify it as another fad.) Any "raw" sugar that you take in on this plan is not only unnecessary but can be deleterious. Your body will get along very nicely doing its own chemical thing. Let it make its own raw elements from the food you eat. Once you get on a sugar kick—whether it be candy, cake, pies, or what have you—you'll find it very difficult to get off. Then you'll feel discouraged and guilty, and motivation to lose weight flies out the window.

Many girls get a severe "sugar craving" just before their period. At such times, they tell me, they can "practically climb the wall" for something sweet. To alleviate this craving, I recommend the fructose preparations that are now available. Fructose is a sugar, it is sweet, it doesn't taste exactly like sugar-sugar (nothing really does), but it will take the edge off your sugar crunch for the time being and it will prevent you from getting into the sugar-binge habit every time your period is due. If you don't like the idea of trying the fructose, eat a piece of fruit to satisfy the sugar craving. If what you are talking about is a real bodily craving, your body will certainly be satisfied with this natural sugar, which was around long before the confectionary industry ever made its appearance. If, however, what you are talking about is a mental craving, that is quite another thing.

"What I really want is a piece of candy when my period is due," one young lady recently confided to me. I assured her that this was not a true sugar craving.

"Oh, yes it is," she insisted. "I eat just about a whole box of chocolates when my period is due. I never eat them at any other time."

I suggested she try a sweet piece of fruit—a cantaloupe or even a peach. She insisted it was candy and nothing else that would help her. But in time, having convinced her to try the fruit, she discovered she really wasn't after the taste of the fruit—it was the taste of the candy itself she wanted. But this was not a bodily demand; candy was not around when the human body was being put together. The very fact that she did not care for the substituted sweet made her aware that what she had been calling a "sugar craving" was really Madison Avenue hype. Once she was convinced of this, and was determined not to let the advertisers get the best of her, the so-called craving for candy before her period disappeared and she was able to lose weight far more effectively. Today she is normal weight, stays away from sugar, and doesn't dare trust herself with even an occasional piece of candy, period or no.

JUNK FOODS

One of the basic misconceptions about junk foods is that they are a source of "empty" calories. This is not always true. A calorie is a measurement of energy, regardless of where it comes from. I mention this because the term "empty calories" has led at least several of my teen patients to assume that such calories would, being empty, do them no harm—an ingenuous, if selective, stretching of the definition. Actually, the term "empty calorie" refers to food having no nutritive value, only supplying the prerequisites for you to get fatter. A lot depends on your definition of junk foods if you want to avoid some and have others. Popcorn is generally considered a junk food, yet by itself, as I have mentioned elsewhere, it is low in calories. The problem, of course, arises with the salt and butter that is sprinkled over it. A nice treat can be arranged with popcorn using a salt substitute and margarine in reasonable quantities. Popcorn will serve the additional purpose of filling you up. Of course, if you take in a quantity of popcorn and then drink several glasses of water, and if you get on the scale shortly thereafter to see how much weight you've lost on your new diet, you may be considerably disappointed. You may, in fact, be horrified to find that you've actually put weight on. But wait a minute before running around the house banging your head against the walls. The popcorn/water mix inside you does weigh something, and until your body passes it, this "dead weight" will contribute to your overall fat weight. It is just another caution to you to use your head when you diet. The top part.

Diet candies, even diet chocolate, usually with the amount of calories on the label, are available. Depending on the manufacturer, they taste to a greater or lesser extent like the real thing, and as long as they do not go down in excess amounts, and as long as they do not merely revive in you the desire for the real thing and have you put this desire into action, they are probably all right to use as "junk food snacks," as one of my patients calls them. Although I have spoken to many doctors who claim they have had considerable success with these items as far as their patients are concerned, I cannot say the same. In a way it is like the fake cigarettes whose function is to get people to stop smoking. The real smokers want the real thing or nothing. As a former "candy freak," I'm afraid I feel the same way regarding my own habit. And most of my patients seem to agree with me. For teens in particular it is awkward, if not impossible, to refuse a proffered piece of candy for the diet substitute they then have to take from purse or pocket. The whole thing is not only too much of a hassle, it's downright embarrassing. The best thing I have found, as far as junk food is concerned, is to avoid it as much as possible. That doesn't mean forever. It means until you have gotten to a more normal weight than you are at present. At that time you will, hopefully, be able to use junk foods as occasional snacks, rather than using them to repeat the process of gaining weight. But if you are the type of person who can't eat one potato chip, one bite of ice cream, a small portion of pie, a reasonable bit of cake, a taste of pudding, a thin slice of pizza—and most of us addicts fall in that category—then I suggest it would be wise of you to make up your mind to avoid these things altogether. Don't consider this as "giving up all those items that make life worth living," as one of my patients recently mourned. Instead look at it the way I put it to her:

"What you really don't want to give up is the most essential item that makes life worth living—being thin. All other items are only secondary to that."

WHY DO GIRLS GET FATTER THAN BOYS?

AVERAGE WEIGHTS FOR BOYS AND GIRLS

| | Boys | | Girls | |
Age (years)	Height (inches)	Weight (pounds)	Height (inches)	Weight (pounds)
12	59	88	60	92
13	62	99	62	102
14	65	112	63	111
15	67	125	64	118
16	68	137	64	123
17	69	146	64	125
18	69	152	65	126

As I mentioned earlier, any weight gain of fat means that the body is taking in more calories than it can handle for its energy requirements. Since the body stores calories, any excess of these substances is then stored as fat. The body stores few substances. It does not store protein, vitamins, hormones, or water. It does store calories. Adolescent boys and girls use up a large number of the calories they ingest in growth. When you are growing, of course, you can thereby take in a large number of calories and not show a weight gain (unless the amount you are taking in is so out of proportion to what your body can conceivably use up that it will store calories even in this instance).

Once they begin menstruating, many girls slow down in their growth, thus requiring fewer calories from that point on than they have been taking in during the period of rapid growth that preceded. However, most girls, not aware of this, continue to eat just as they did before, seeing no necessity to cut down or change their eating habits, since they never had a weight problem. Suddenly, as such a girl, you are horrified to find that you are putting on weight.

Boys, however, not having a menstrual cycle to contend with, continue to grow fairly rapidly up to age nineteen, in some cases longer, and can continue taking in calories at the same rate as before, since the energy thus furnished to the body is being used up in actual girth rather than fat. That is the main reason why, being a girl, you can contend with a boy in school or on the ballfield, at social events and even in the military—but you cannot contend with him on a calorie basis. This difference is not only one of adolescence. It continues throughout life. Men, in general, can almost always take off weight more rapidly than women, given the same age and body structure. Men, of course, even after the teen period is long over, can always eat more than women, since they have more muscle and bone to feed.

I go into this at some length because I have found an unfortunate tendency for boys and girls to compete with one another in the weight-loss game. Whether it be boyfriend or brother, husband or cousin, don't run a race, as a woman, with any man when it comes to losing weight. In my own practice, I have had to separate husbands and wives from coming into the weighing room together. Almost invariably the husband will lose more than the wife, who will then complain about how good she was and how much he cheated. It doesn't pay. Rapidity of weight loss is one aspect where, like it or not, sexual partiality shows through to the woman's disadvantage.

How rapidly, then, can you lose? This is hard to say. I know I could make a big hit with you at this time by saying that if you follow my plan you can lose two pounds a day. Unfortunately, not only would I be lying to you, but to lose that kind of weight would be unhealthy.

HOW FAST CAN I LOSE?

The average amount of weight that is considered healthy and medically sound to lose each week is about 3,500 calories' worth.

That is one pound.

All right, I can hear you complaining, one pound? Is that all I'm going to lose? Only one pound a week?

Well, how much would you like to lose?

I'll be reasonable, you say. How about a pound a day?

Of course, you might really consider that reasonable. And there are diet plans around that will tell you that in the first week (they are generally careful to so specify) you can lose seven pounds or ten pounds or fourteen pounds. The fact is that when we are talking about this kind of weight loss we are generally speaking about water loss. But that's all right with you, isn't it? After all, weight is weight. (Even these plans don't pretend you'll continue to lose that kind of weight.)

Well, calm down. There is no way in the world you will lose the kind of weight you are talking of on a consistent basis. On my plan you will lose in the neighborhood of two pounds per week. And you'll be happy with that kind of loss because you will realize that such a loss is a lot of weight for several reasons:

1. You will no longer be gaining weight—so you'll be reversing a process that has probably been haunting you for a while.
2. You will not be staying at the same weight. How long has it been since you have been off the routine of gaining a pound, losing a pound—and averaging out at about the same top weight week after week? Oh, you say to yourself, If I could only establish a downward pattern! Well, now you will be doing just that.
3. You will actually be losing weight week after week. So this is the final plus factor—if I may call it that. You will be losing. If you lose a half a pound in a week, that's just fine. Never say to yourself, "Oh, all I lost is . . ." Once you start with that phrase, you are already defeated. It doesn't matter if you add to it ten pounds or twenty pounds. No matter how you end that particular sentence you are a loser—but not in the sense that you want to be. Once you start by saying, "All I lost is . . ." it doesn't matter how much you lost. It will never be enough. Don't face that particular putdown. Instead, start by saying, "It's wonderful. This week I lost a

pound." Or two pounds. Or three pounds. See what I mean? You are being positive, you are taking an approach that is self-congratulatory and that will ensure further success. Sound simple? Maybe so. All I can tell you is that it works. And if something works, that should be good enough. I've seen the success of this plan on thousands of patients in over sixteen years of treating overweight individuals. These are people just like you. In fact, it can be you. All you have to do is set your mind to it.

So don't worry about how fast you can lose. Rest assured that you *will* lose. That you *will* be slim. And put your energies toward following the plan rather than in running a race. If you will do that much for yourself, I'll do the rest for you.

WHAT ABOUT FASTING?

Short-term fasts are popular with adolescents—at least, that has been my experience. However, I do not feel that such fasts allow your body adequate time to adapt efficiently enough to use up stored fat. There are other factors involved as well.

For one thing, going on a fast for more than one day can result in making you tired and irritable and disturb your powers of concentration—especially in school. I don't think this is a good thing for people in your age group. Besides, all too often a fasting teen feels, once the fast is over, that he or she has everything coming because of the self-denial he or she has imposed. Then comes the eating binge. This starve-binge pattern, previously discussed, which involves days of fasting followed by days of overconsumption (even though you may not consider it as such), is not the best thing in the world for your body. Add to this the ancillary methods that teens have told me they use in a desperate attempt to get the weight off—such as vomiting after eating or the use of laxatives—and a real problem can develop. These are not the eating habits that I want to develop in you, nor, I am sure, are they ones you would feel particularly comfortable with. Even if you eat enough to avoid the symptoms of anorexia, this sort of treatment, rising directly out of the false philosophy of fasting, can end you up in a heap of trouble.

In a word then, forget the word "fast." Forget about losing "fast" and forget about fasting to lose. Instead, consider at length. Consider how long this problem has been with you. Consider thoroughly what you want to do about yourself, what kind of a person you are and how you can adapt yourself to a reasonable, medically sound weight loss plan. If you cannot do this, forget about losing weight. You are the same person fat as thin. If this is unacceptable, fine. Now you have to make a choice between losing your mind or losing your weight. All these fad-diet, quick-weight-loss plans will do is frustrate you beyond measure. You will end up totally enraged—and just as fat as ever. Why not avoid this right at the beginning and follow a reasonable plan? In the long run, you won't have any choice *but* to do this. Why not do it to begin with?

TIPS FOR SUCCESSFUL DIETING

It is advisable to have some idea as to how many calories you are taking in. If you wish, you can actually sit down and figure them out. On an average (and please remember that you are not an average but an individual), the total daily caloric intake for teenage girls can be between 1,400 to 1,800 calories and for boys between 1,700 to 2,200 calories. You can take in less than this, but any dieting must be done under the supervision of a doctor who is treating you personally.

Avoid all sugar and all things of which sugar is a part. You know what these items are as well as I do; there is very little sense my listing them here. Either you will avoid them or you won't. If you don't avoid them all, avoid as many as you can. No one is perfect. It is better to admit to yourself, "Yes, I fouled up, but I will try again tomorrow," than to say, "I did it again. There's no hope for me." There is always hope—especially if you don't try to be a saint. Once you tell yourself you have to be perfect, all you are doing is looking to fail. Maybe this is what you want—another good excuse to call yourself names, to go off your diet, to stay fat. If this is the case, better you find it out now and enjoy the rest of your life as a fat person. But hopefully this isn't what you want. What you really want is to be thin. Just don't get so up tight about it that you are constantly calling yourself names.

Eat at least one fresh fruit a day. On occasion you can eat two. You should eat these substances slowly and enjoy them. Don't gobble them down as some sort of duty. Make them last. Once you get used to taking your "sweet" this way, you will get to look forward to it. It may seem deranged of me to say so, but you can actually get to feel about your fruit as you have felt in the past about candy, or ice cream or whatever your particular pet treat may have been. It isn't particularly difficult to bring this about. What you must do to make it work is to make a habit out of your fruit pattern. It will then take hold pretty quickly on its own.

Eat about half a cup of raw and/or cooked vegetables daily. You will find this, for the most part, on your diet cycle in the next chapter. I suggest that vegetables be cooked in a wok. That way they are somewhere between raw and cooked. They are also mighty tasty. If you have not been a vegetable eater in the past, cooking these items in a wok will make you one. Try this yourself, or ask whoever prepares the meals in your family to try it for you. I run into many teens who have difficulty eating many vegetables. Wok cooking almost invariably solves this problem.

Because an over-indulgence in fat and fatty foods can lead to problems as you get older, it is a good idea to limit your intake of meats and other proteins that are high in fat. Included in this list are cold cuts, sausage, red meat, and many of the hard cheeses. This still leaves you quite a lot to eat, so don't start feeling bad. I'm not cutting these items out—but I'm not really adding them in, either. They form the "gray area" boundary line between what you should be doing to lose your weight, and what you actually may do in practice.

Limit your intake of butter, fats, oils, and all such products. This is the same reason as given above. Teenagers generally eat far too much of these substances. Not only do they add pounds to you, but they interfere with complexion, skin tone, and possibly hormone balance. As a girl, you don't need any of these complications.

Don't cut out carbohydrates. You will find on your diet cycle cereals, breads, and other starches. These are necessary to help you maintain good health. All too often the teenager will get involved in an "all or nothing" approach to dieting. As I keep stressing throughout the course of this book, that is not the way to achieve long-term success in the weight-losing game.

Drink 8 eight-ounce glasses of water a day. Water is critical—as I keep saying. I would like to say it once again here. Certainly the water is more important than soda. It is even more important than juice. For some reason, we are all tied up in knots about fruit juice. I have never been able to find out why. There is nothing magical about fruit juice—it will *not* cure a cold, will not help avoid pregnancy, will not provide you with all the vitamins and minerals you need, will not help you lose weight. All your drinking of juice will do is help the fruit juice industry. They are rich enough; you don't have to help them any more. Better you should start helping yourself by drinking water. You may substitute seltzer or Perrier water for some of your water if you wish.

Take a general vitamin (multivitamin) and mineral supplement every day.

Avoid fad diets and all imbalanced diets. That is, those plans that involve eating only a few food groups to the exclusion of all others.

If you are going to fast, don't do it for more than a day. Remember, this is an artificial way to lose weight; it can hardly be sustained or made into a long-term habit. And then, if you are like most people, you will likely make up for your fast by eating twice as much the next day. Hopefully you won't, of course, and then the fasting can do you some good. But one day is enough.

Do not take any pills to help you lose weight without being under the care of your doctor. Certainly you should not take any of your friends' pills—which is done more frequently than you might imagine. It is all too easy to pop a pill from a friend who claims miracles for it. It is all too easy to go to the drugstore and pick up any of the commercial preparations "guaranteed" to make you lose weight. There is no such thing as a pill that will make you lose weight. The best that such medications can do for you is to feed your fantasy that you don't have to do the job for yourself; the worst is that they may make you sick. Certainly, in the end, they will get you discouraged. Feeding a fantasy is as disastrous as overfeeding your body. In the final analysis, the only pill that will help you lose weight is—and I'll say it again— the one situated on top of your neck. Learn to use that one—by gradually but firmly changing your eating habits.

Don't be misled by advertising promises. These have mushroomed lately, not only as "special pills for quick weight loss" or "rapid weight loss pills—no diet necessary," but in the form of special "clinics," many of whom specialize merely in taking your or your parents' money. Any medicine or clinic that tells you it can make fat disappear in some magical fashion should be suspect. Once again, I repeat that the only way you can get rid of your fat is by eating it. This involves taking less food in and burning up, as well, the excess that is there. In order to do this you must work at it. Perhaps you don't like to be told that. Nevertheless, it is true. No diet alone can do the job, even mine. Only you can do the job—by taking the losing game step by step and learning when you are hungry and when you are not.

It's that simple. And that effective.

10

The Teenage Five-Day Cycle

If you are in your late teens, say sixteen to twenty years, you've probably already experienced a growth spurt and are now at a stage where you can expect relatively little increase in height. In general, a girl's growth spurt comes at an earlier age than a boy's. Of course, there are "early" developers and "late" developers, and if you are uncertain whether or not you have a lot more growing to do, you should check with your doctor.

The Teenage Five-Day Cycle is geared to those of you in your late teens whose growth rates have slowed down and who therefore require fewer calories. This plan provides between 900 and 1,100 calories per day, whereas the Basic Menu Plan in Chapter 8 allows for between 1,200 and 1,500 calories.

WEIGHT LOSS IMMEDIATELY

The Teenage Five-Day Cycle is an attempt to come to immediate grips with your weight problem. It is meant to start you off so the weight loss you achieve will be quickly measurable. What you want, of course, is results. At this time of your life, probably having tried many other diets in the past, you are looking for something that will begin to work immediately, that will keep you comfortable, that is structured so it can easily be followed during the course of your normal activities, and that will help you, once you lose weight, to keep it off.

DON'T WORRY ABOUT YOUR BODY SIZE

Many overweight and most obese teenagers tend to overestimate their body size. It's easy to exaggerate a fault—and better you should do it before someone else does. However, your body size should not affect how well you will do in this weight-loss program. Girls, especially, tend to overestimate body widths such as waists, hips, chest (some underestimate here), and even faces. The heavier you get, the more you overestimate and the more unattractive you end up considering yourself. However, it may be quite a relief to you to find out that your own estimate of how you look—"like a camel," "like an elephant," "like I'm wearing flesh-colored jodhpurs" are some of the self-descriptive phrases I've heard—will not adversely affect your weight loss on this plan. In studies that have been done, no significant correlation was found between body attitude and accuracy in following a specific diet to lose weight. I had always thought that patients who overestimate their body width took a negative attitude that would color the results of their weight-loss endeavor. This does not seem to be the case. As one investigator of the subject has written, "Weight loss is not affected by how accurate the patients were in estimating their own body images or in how they felt about their bodies."

So, if you want to keep insulting yourself, do so—for some people this is a motivating factor. But at least insult yourself reasonably.

KEEPING A LOW PROFILE AT SCHOOL

"How am I to stay on my diet at school?" is a constant question.

My answer: "Easily."

Consider. The only meal that falls into school hours is lunch. The only snack is the midmorning one. As far as lunch is concerned, any of the items mentioned can be packed in a lunch-box. Stay away from the lunch counter at school. That doesn't mean you should tell your friends you are trying to lose weight. The fewer people that know about this the better. Make up any excuse you wish—for example, tell your friends you have an allergy problem that your doctor is trying to solve. Or, if it comes to that, eat by yourself. There shouldn't be all that much difficulty about it.

As for the midmorning snack, you should have some free time during the course of the morning to enjoy this treat. But don't make an issue of it. If you can't manage it for one or two days, better to do without it. Do not add it to your afternoon meal on the basis that you have it coming. Disregard it if for some reason you do not get to eat it.

Above all, treat yourself and your diet with respect. Remember, you may feel foolish at first being "different" from your friends, but this is a feeling you simply have to get over. Your problem is not their problem; in the long run they don't care about you. Hopefully you will care more about yourself than they do.

INTAKE VERSUS OUTPUT

For a long time it was taken as axiomatic that teens of both sexes, though perhaps boys more than girls, consumed roughly the same amount of calories as did nonobese teens but were more lethargic when it came to spending them. In other words, fat people are lazier than thin ones, since they have more to carry around; this makes them spend fewer calories, which, added to the *normal* amount of food they are taking in, makes them even fatter.

Many doctors still believe this to be a primary factor in obese teens.

I do not believe this to be the case.

In a recent study of a number of families each with an obese and a nonobese male child, it was shown that the obese boys consumed more calories by far than did their nonobese brothers. The obese boys also tended to eat much faster. In general, the obese children were far less active than their nonobese brothers inside their homes, were slightly less active outside their homes, and were equally active at school.

However, and here's the truly interesting part, when activity values were converted into energy expenditure by measurement of oxygen consumption, the obese boys expended *more* calories in moving than did their brothers. As a result, there was no difference in energy expenditure between obese and nonobese boys outside the home and at school.

These findings are contrary to observations in adults, which indicate little difference in food intake between obese and nonobese persons. Also, obese adults may not always eat more rapidly than nonobese adults. (This is contrary to my own experience in the matter.)

This study casts doubt on earlier reports that obese children are physically inactive. Only at home, and only when caloric expenditure was ignored, could obese boys be considered inactive. At home, and at their most inactive time, obese boys expended as many calories as their nonobese brothers, and in outdoor activities they actually expended more calories.

Obesity in these boys is thus maintained by increased caloric intake rather than by decreased caloric output. While the study does not indicate how these boys became obese, results strongly suggest a similar dynamic.

The above report, by Drs. Waxman and Stunkard, was printed in a recent issue of the *Journal of Pediatrics*. Many of my fat teens will be glad to see in cold print what they have been maintaining all along—that they are not slothful, inert, lazy; that they don't just lie around all day. In fact, as one of them put it to me in a succinct manner, "I must sweat half of myself away each day." What the above study shows is that such an individual eats back the half and more of himself that he does sweat off. This does not mean that exercise in any of the ways usually proposed does not apply to you or that it isn't important. Not at all. It does show that it simply isn't enough, that what you need is to take in fewer calories. In this regard, let us take a look at the Five-Day Cycle and see how it can help start you off. Although this is similar to the adolescent cycle, there are fewer calories overall to make up for the slower growth rate.

A HEAD START ON THE BATTLE: SUGGESTED MENU OUTLINE

None of these foods *must* be eaten. At least three hours *must* elapse between meals. At least 1½ hours *must* elapse between meals and snacks.

A.M.	4 ounces fruit or juice 1 egg 2 ounces meat ½ slice whole-wheat bread or 1 cup hot or cold cereal
MIDMORNING PICKUP (OPTIONAL)	1 cup skim milk 2 ounces meat
NOON	3 ounces meat 1 cup vegetables (mostly leafy) 1 tablespoon any oil
MIDAFTERNOON PICKUP	1 apple or similar fruit 1 cup skim milk
P.M.	4 ounces fish or fowl 1 cup legumes 1 cup vegetable 1 slice whole-wheat bread or 1 small potato
EVENING SNACK	½ cup plain yogurt 1 orange

The above is, as stated, merely an outline. The following five-day plan will play variations on it. You may, yourself, vary it within limits.

USING THE FIVE-DAY CYCLE

I have used a five-day plan for teenagers because I especially want you kids off the "weekend special." I don't want you to keep thinking of the weekend as a special sort of time when you can let loose. I want you to get into the habit of rotating your five days and stop asking yourself, "What's new? What can I eat today to celebrate?" I'll give you something to celebrate—getting thin. And here's how you accomplish it. The Five-Day Cycle is approximately 800 to 1,000 calories per day and I have varied these to get the best results. Vegetables may be steamed or stir-fried.

DAY 1

BREAKFAST
½ cup fresh or canned orange juice
2 pieces melba toast
1 cup skim milk
Coffee, tea

LUNCH
½ cup cottage cheese
Salad (½ cup diced peaches, ½ cup diced pears, ½ cup celery, lettuce)

DINNER
4 ounces breast of chicken
1 cup celery and green pepper
½ cup cooked brussels sprouts
1 cup cooked carrots
1 cup skim milk

BEDTIME
1 cup plain yogurt

DAY 2

BREAKFAST
½ grapefruit
1 thin slice whole-wheat bread

1 egg, boiled or poached
Coffee, tea

LUNCH

⅓ cup cottage cheese
Salad (½ cup escarole, ½ cup cabbage, ½ cup green pepper, ½ cup celery) with lemon juice dressing
1 can diet soda

DINNER

4 ounces broiled fillet of sole
½ cup cooked beets
4 ounces eggplant, sliced and fried in nonstick pan
3 slices tomato
½ cup unsweetened fruit cocktail
Coffee, tea

BEDTIME

1 cup skim milk

DAY 3

BREAKFAST

1 orange
⅔ cup puffed wheat cereal
1 cup skim milk (may use part for cereal)
Coffee, tea

LUNCH

4 ounces cooked crabmeat
Salad (½ cup celery, ½ cup lettuce, ½ cup tomato) with lemon juice dressing
½ cup carrot sticks

DINNER

4 ounces raw clams or boiled shrimp
4 ounces broiled haddock
½ cup cabbage
½ cup turnips
½ cup brussels sprouts
Coffee, tea

BEDTIME	1 cup skim milk

Day 4

BREAKFAST	1 orange 1 egg, boiled or poached 1 regular slice whole-wheat toast ½ cup corn flakes Coffee, tea
LUNCH	½ cup cottage cheese 4-ounce hamburger, no bun 3 slices tomato 1 can diet soda
DINNER	4 ounces breast of chicken 1 cup cooked broccoli ½ cup baked potato 1 baked apple, no sugar
BEDTIME	1 cup skim milk

Day 5

BREAKFAST	½ cup orange juice 1 piece melba toast 1 cup skim milk Coffee, tea
LUNCH	⅓ cup cottage cheese 4 ounces boiled shrimp ½ cucumber 1 piece melba toast 1 can diet soda
DINNER	4 ounces boiled lobster 3 slices tomato ½ cup green pepper 1 slice whole-wheat bread ½ grapefruit Coffee, tea

BEDTIME   1 cup skim milk

As you have probably noticed, there is quite a bit less food on the Five-Day Cycle than on the Basic Menu Plan in Chapter 8. However, if you feel on a particular day that you could really use a little more food, you may switch to the Basic Menu Plan for a day or so. You may do this on a regular basis if you wish. Of course, you will lose faster by staying with the Five-Day Cycle.

This brings us to the weekends.

HOW TO HANDLE THE WEEKENDS

Weekends are usually more difficult to lose weight on than are weekdays. Most people are fairly used to a rather disciplined existence during the week; during the weekend they tend to feel more relaxed and freer, the tendency being to let things slide rather than pay attention to a routine. There is no reason you shouldn't feel that way as well. So I have devised a different sort of plan for you to follow during this time. It will only involve your asking yourself, over and over when the urge strikes you to eat: "Am I hungry?" If the answer is "Yes," then there will be plenty for you to eat—though, hopefully, you will be eating differently than you did when you got yourself fat. That is: slowly, only when hungry and at no other time, not considering special foods for special times of the day, not eating just because the clock tells you it is breakfast or lunch or dinner time. You will notice that I rarely associate food with these words, preferring to note an eating time by some other word. It is all part of the learning process that I hope you will faithfully follow. Here, then is your weekend eating plan.

FRUITS FOR NIBBLING

These nibbling foods are for satisfying the feelings of hunger that you may get throughout the day. Such feelings will come at irregular, not regular, intervals. They may not come for long periods of time, or they may come at short ones. These foods, together with your knowledge of how to eat them as previously mentioned, will more than keep your stomach content. Do not exceed the amounts given. You may have all or none of these items per day as you see fit.

> ½ grapefruit *or* ⅓ cantaloupe *or* a 3-inch slice of other melon *or* a whole orange (no watermelon— too much sugar)
> 1 raw apple *or* 1 raw pear
> ½ cup strawberries
> ⅓ cup unsweetened fruit cocktail

On the above items you may have any or all of these fruits. In other words, you may have ½ grapefruit, 1 apple, ½ cup strawberries, and ⅓ cup unsweetened fruit cocktail if you wish. If you don't want all that, don't eat all that. You cannot add to one day, however, those items you did not eat from the day before.

VEGETABLES FOR NIBBLING

> 1 large carrot
> 2 stalks celery
> ½ medium onion
> 1 small tomato
> ½ cup of lettuce *or* ½ cup cucumber *or* ½ cup spinach
> ½ cup mushrooms *or* ½ cup cauliflower

Although I ask that the above foods be eaten preferably raw, stir-frying is fine. (You may also have the onion fried if a non-stick pan is used, no butter.) I just don't want to have mush made out of the vegetables. It's hard to chew mush.

SOUPS

> ½ cup of any jellied clear soup *or* 1 cup of bouillon, consommé, *or* any clear soup with a minimum of fat

MUST FOODS

Although all the foods listed so far may or may not be eaten on a regular or irregular basis depending on your hunger, this category, the "must" foods should be taken on a regular basis, divided three times during the day. These are foods fairly rich in potassium, a mineral I'd like to supply you with. I'd rather you got your potassium in this manner than in pill form. These foods are also meant to satisfy that "sweet tooth" that may inconveniently otherwise occur, and the prunes, at least, will help keep you regular.

"Must" foods involve 3 dried prunes *or* 3 dried apricot halves *or* a 1-inch slice of cranberry sauce, all divided through the day. The cranberry sauce should be cut in thirds. You may combine any of these items if you wish, taking 1 portion of each at the stated intervals through the day.

I, personally, prefer the prunes over the others. Dried prunes—with pits. Not the depitted variety the food industry serves up so that the entire mess resembles one large prune that one can readily dive into. You will chew your dried prune with pit more carefully than the depitted variety—you don't want to break your teeth, after all. And when you have done nibbling the meat away from the pit you have a calculated pacifier in your mouth that you can chase with your tongue, tuck in a corner of your cheek, suck on—and if you get into an argument, you've got a weapon. The prune pit is, therefore, an essential tool.

WATER

As noted throughout this book, water is critical. For the sake of completeness I will reiterate here that you must drink 8 eight-ounce glasses of water each day, divided throughout the day. This is essential. I prefer the water be cold, though it need not be ice cold. Anyone can drink water; it's easy. Kids tell me, "I'll never get all that water down. It gets stuck." As though you've got some sort of pocket in the throat. But all the soda and milkshakes go down; the pocket doesn't interfere with them. A peculiar pocket—more in your head than in your throat.

PROTEIN FOODS

Beef
Lamb
Veal
Fresh ham
Pork roast or chops
Fresh fish
Canned fish (tuna, salmon; preferably water packed)
Shellfish (shrimp, clams, lobster on occasion, mussels, oysters, crabs; no butter sauce)
Chicken (very little skin)
Turkey (no skin)
Liver (either beef or pork)
Frankfurters or chicken frankfurters (maximum 3 a week; divide them up)
Do not eat:
Smoked fish or meats
Salted meats such as ham, prosciutto, bacon, etc.
Fatty meats or fish (mackerel, bluefish)

Trim fat from meat to a great extent.

You can have your protein foods prepared just about any way you like. It is best *not* to have it deep-fat fried or breaded. Almost any other way is fine.

How much of these protein foods can you eat? That is really up to you. As you can see, I have not provided you with any specific measurement here—because I have no idea how hungry you will be. And it is your hunger that will make all the difference as to the amounts that you eat. Now, this is rather a sophisticated manner of approaching the problem, but I certainly think you are old enough to manage such a grown-up approach. What do I really mean? I mean that you may have these protein foods in *small amounts* as often as you feel truly hungry. That means, no meals. No breakfast, lunch, or dinner. You may eat once a day, you may eat five times a day. If you are truly hungry, that is.

But let us say you are truly hungry. You say to yourself, "Boy, today I could eat a horse!" Well, fine. Start with a colt. If you think you could eat a dozen hamburgers, start with one. A whole chicken? Start with a single thigh or breast. A twelve-ounce steak? Start with four ounces. Then, after you have eaten what is on your plate, slowly, enjoying it, sit back and ask yourself again, Am I still hungry? If the answer is no, then you are done. If the answer is, honestly, yes, then take some more. The idea is not to put a whole lot on your plate—because if you do, you will end up eating it, hungry or not. That is what you have always done, if you stop to think about it.

Actually, pausing after you have finished what is on your plate and asking yourself if you need more is a good break in the eating pattern. It is like getting a telephone call in the middle of a meal. You know, there you are, eating, and the phone rings. You get up to answer it, interrupting the eating cycle, and when you go to sit down again, you aren't as hungry as you were before. You sort of have to start all over again with the food. It is just possible you may not be hungry now. At least give yourself the option.

DAIRY FOODS

You may have 1 egg every day, either hard-boiled or poached. I suggest this method of cooking the egg rather than frying or scrambling or soft-boiling, since there is more substance to the egg. Even poached it provides more satiety to your mouth. There is more to chew. After all, how long does it take you to eat a soft-boiled egg? Zoom—and it's gone. And now you are looking around for something to eat. With a hard-boiled egg you can really have a meal. Cut it into several pieces and eat it with your fingers. Eating with your fingers gets you closer to the food than does eating with a fork. You can better appreciate the food. That's what eating is all about—appreciating food. Up to now the communication has all been one way—down the hatch. Now you are going to spend time trying to break that habit of simply eating with your mouth. You are going to eat with your nose, with your eyes, with your sense of anticipation, with your sense of aesthetics. You are going to have a relationship with your food instead of taking it for granted. The wider you open your mouth, interestingly enough, the more satiety you get. You can fool your mouth in this way, make it think there's more going in than has actually gone. That will tend to satisfy the "mouth hunger," which, in fact, is why most people eat. Roll up a piece of hard-boiled egg in a lettuce leaf; now you have a sandwich. You have to open your mouth fairly wide to get it in. You'll be surprised how nicely this will help to satisfy your mouth hunger. If you satisfy your mouth hunger, your stomach hunger will take care of itself. Remember, a good part of the trick is to eat slowly.

You may have 1 glass of low fat or skim milk daily.

You may have ½ cup plain yogurt as an extra treat if you wish.

BEVERAGES

You may have as much as you wish of the following except for diet soda. I have limited diet soda to no more than 2 cans a day. Diet soda is quite salty and, for many kids, only serves to keep them in the soda-drinking habit—which is one of the habits I am trying to break you of.

All of the following are fine:

> Coffee (no sugar; 2 teaspoons of
> skim milk per cup. You may use
> any of the artificial powdered
> milks)
> Postum
> Tea
> Carbonated water
> Mineral water
> Seltzer
> Diet soda (as stated above)

SUGAR SUBSTITUTES

I would like to put in a brief word here regarding these substances. For my own part, I do not use them, since I find that the main purpose they serve is to keep my taste for sugar alive. I understand that many people swear by them—as a direct alternative to sugar. Let me give you a word of advice: If you can do without these substances it would be far better to do so. All they do is remind you of what you really want. I have the same problem with diet candy—as I have mentioned before. At the same time, I am not going to put myself in the position of forbidding these items to you. But I would certainly suggest that you use them with caution.

With this word of caution, you may use saccharin or sucaryl calcium. Try to stay away from the sucaryl sodium, which contains rather a lot of the element sodium, which will make your body retain water.

SEASONINGS

The following can be used in whatever amounts you like:

>Chives
>Cinnamon (and all other spices)
>Dill
>Horseradish
>Lemon juice (fruit sections or slices as well)
>Lime juice (fruit sections or slices as well)
>Mint
>Mustard
>Onion or garlic powder (*not* garlic salt)
>Paprika
>Pepper (all varieties)
>Peppers (red or green, as seasoning)

Pimiento (as seasoning or for
   color)
Salt substitutes
Sauces (prepared, such as
   Worcestershire, A-1, Tabasco,
   etc; don't overuse because of
   salt content)
Ketchup (use as a condiment only,
   not as a soup; it is high in sugar)
Vinegar
Garlic

The idea for weekend is substitution. It works very well, provided you know what to substitute for what. You won't be hungry, you will be able to eat interesting things—but you will be substituting foods with lower caloric content for the foods you might otherwise be eating. Let us look at some of these substitutions and how many calories you can save while still having a good time. This is kind of a game you can play—certainly better than the Russian roulette you are playing now.

For example, let's forget about dieting and compare a "typical" meal with its substitutes. This will show you the principles involved. For an overall view, we will look at an entire day's worth of food:

Regular	Calories	Substitute	Calories
BREAKFAST			
½ glass orange juice	50	½ glass orange juice	50
1 scrambled egg	120	1 boiled egg	78
2 slices bacon	100	1 slice bacon	50
2 pats butter	100	Low-calorie margarine	34
2 cups coffee, each with 2 lumps sugar, 2 tablespoons cream	220	2 cups coffee, with artificial sweetener, non-fat dry milk	22
Total calories	786		304

Regular	Calories	Substitute	Calories
MIDMORNING SNACK			
1 cup coffee with 2 lumps sugar, 2 tablespoons cream	110	1 cup coffee with artificial sweetener and nonfat dry milk	11
1 small Danish pastry	140	2 low-calorie cookies	50
Total calories	250		61
LUNCH			
Hamburger (3 ounces) on bun	350	Hamburger (3 ounces) on bun	350
1 slice apple pie	338	Low-calorie pudding	123
1 cup whole milk	165	1 cup skim milk	80
Total calories	853		553
MIDAFTERNOON SNACK			
8 ounces cola beverage	105	1 cup low-calorie soda	2
1 custard (4-ounce cup)	205	2 low-calorie cookies	50
Total calories	310		52
DINNER			
½ cup tomato juice	25	Consommé (1 cup)	10
6 ounces meat loaf with ¼ cup gravy	680	6-ounce lean broiled club steak	320
½ cup mashed potatoes	123	1 medium baked potato	100
½ cup green peas	72	12 spears asparagus	40

Regular	Calories	Substitute	Calories
2 slices French bread with 2 pats butter	260	2 slices French bread with 2 pats low-calorie margarine	34
Tossed salad with 1½ tablespoons Roquefort cheese dressing	170	Hearts of lettuce with low-calorie dressing	35
Iced plain layer cake	290	1 cup low-calorie whipped dessert	123
1 cup coffee with 2 lumps sugar and 2 tablespoons cream	110	1 cup coffee with artificial sweetener and nonfat dry milk	11
Total calories	1,894		673
Total calories for day	4,093		1,643

A saving of 2,380 calories

Now this should give you a pretty good idea of how to eat over the weekends. Remember that substituting one food for another only works if you watch the size of your portions. If you eat a bigger portion of the substitute food than you should, you won't be saving the calories you should. *There should be no such thing as a second helping.* What you are after is first aid—not second helpings. Just to give you an idea of what is available and how you can use it, you might study the following list of items and use them to your advantage. This will allow you to personalize your menus over the weekend. *You don't have to eat three meals a day if you don't feel you need them.* Study the lists I have provided you in the following pages and make up your own menu plans based on them and the number of calories you feel you need each day:

Begin right now correcting your portion size and start substituting foods from column B for foods in column A:

Column A	Calories	Column B	Calories
BEVERAGES			
Milk (whole, 1 cup)	165	Milk (skim, 1 cup)	80
Prune juice (1 cup)	170	Tomato juice (1 cup)	50
Soft drink (1 cup)	105	Diet drink (1 cup)	1
Coffee (2 tablespoons cream and 2 lumps sugar)	110	Coffee (black with artificial sweetener)	0
Cocoa (all-milk; 1 cup)	235	Cocoa (milk and water, 1 cup)	140
Chocolate malted milkshake (1 cup)	500	Sweetened lemonade (1 cup)	100
BREAKFAST FOODS			
Rice flakes (1 cup)	110	Puffed rice (1 cup)	50
Eggs, scrambled (2)	220	Eggs, boiled or poached (2)	160
BUTTER AND CHEESE			
Butter on toast	170	Apple butter on toast	90
Cheese (bleu, cheddar, cream, Swiss; 1 ounce)	105	Cheese (cottage, uncreamed; 1 ounce)	25
DESSERTS			
Angel food cake (2-inch piece)	110	Cantaloupe (½ melon)	40
Cheesecake (2-inch piece)	200	Watermelon (½-inch slice)	60
Chocolate cake and icing (2-inch piece)	425	Sponge cake (2-inch slice)	120

Column A	Calories	Column B	Calories
Fruit cake (2-inch piece)	115	Grapes (1 cup)	65
Pound cake (1-ounce piece)	140	Plums (2)	50
Cupcake with white icing	230	Cupcake (plain)	115
Cookies, assorted (3-inch diameter; 1 piece)	120	Vanilla wafer (dietetic; 1 piece)	25
Ice cream, (½ cup)	150	Yogurt (flavored, ½ cup)	60
Apple pie (1 piece)	345	Tangerine	40
Blueberry pie (1 piece)	290	Blueberries (½ cup)	45
Cherry pie (1 piece)	355	Cherries (½ cup)	40
Custard pie (1 piece)	280	Banana (small)	85
Lemon meringue pie (1 piece)	305	Lemon-flavored gelatin (½ cup)	70
Peach pie (1 piece)	280	Peach	35
Rhubarb pie (1 piece)	265	Grapefruit (½)	55
Rice pudding (½ cup)	140	Pudding, dietetic, nonfat milk (½ cup)	60

FISH AND FOWL

Tuna (canned, oil-packed, 3 ounces)	165	Crabmeat (canned, water-packed, 3 ounces)	80
Oysters, (fried; 6)	400	Raw oysters (in shell and with sauce; 6)	100
Ocean perch, fried (4 ounces)	260	Bass, broiled (4 ounces)	105
Fish sticks (5 sticks, or 4 ounces)	200	Swordfish, broiled (3 ounces)	140

Column A	Calories	Column B	Calories
Lobster meat (4 ounces, 2 teaspoons butter)	300	Lobster meat (4 ounces, lemon)	95
Duck, roasted (3 ounces)	310	Chicken, roasted (3 ounces)	160

MEATS

Column A	Calories	Column B	Calories
Beef loin roast (3 ounces)	290	Pot roast, round (3 ounces)	160
Beef rump roast (3 ounces)	290	Beef rib roast (3 ounces)	200
Swiss steak (3½ ounces)	300	Liver, fried (2½ ounces)	210
Hamburger, regular broiled (3 ounces)	240	Hamburger, lean, broiled (3 ounces)	145
Porterhouse steak (3 ounces)	250	Club steak (3 ounces)	160
Rib lamb chop (3 ounces)	300	Lamb leg roast (3 ounces)	160
Pork chop (3 ounces)	340	Veal chop (3 ounces)	185
Pork roast (3 ounces)	310	Veal roast (3 ounces)	230
Pork sausage (3 ounces)	405	Ham, boiled, lean (3 ounces)	200

POTATOES

Column A	Calories	Column B	Calories
Fried (1 cup)	480	Baked (2- to 3-inch diameter)	100
Mashed (1 cup)	245	Boiled (2- to 3-inch diameter)	100

SALADS

Column A	Calories	Column B	Calories
Green salad with 1 tablespoon oil dressing	180	Green salad with diet dressing	40

Column A	Calories	Column B	Calories
SALADS			
Green salad with 1 tablespoon mayonnaise	125		
Green salad with 1 tablespoon Roquefort, bleu cheese, Russian, or French dressing	105		
SANDWICHES			
Club	375	Bacon and tomato (open)	200
Peanut butter and jelly	275	Egg salad (open)	165
Turkey with 2 tablespoons gravy	520	Hamburger, lean (3 ounces; ½ bun)	200
SNACKS			
Fudge (1 ounce)	115	Vanilla wafers, dietetic (2)	50
Peanuts, salted (1 ounce)	170	Apple	100
Peanuts, roasted (1 cup shelled)	1,375	Grapes (1 cup)	65
Potato chips (10 medium)	115	Pretzels (10 small sticks)	35
Chocolate (1-ounce bar)	145	Marshmallows, toasted (3)	75
SOUPS			
Creamed (1 cup)	210	Chicken noodle (1 cup)	110
Bean (1 cup)	190	Beef noodle (1 cup)	110
Minestrone (1 cup)	105	Beef bouillon (1 cup)	10

Column A	Calories	Column B	Calories
VEGETABLES (cup for cup, boiled or steamed)			
Baked beans	320	Green beans	30
Lima beans	160	Asparagus	30
Corn (canned)	185	Cauliflower	30
Peas (canned)	145	Peas (fresh)	115
Winter squash	75	Summer squash	30
Succotash	260	Spinach	40

These items are, of course, only suggestions. It is not difficult to find substitution items of your own once you get the idea. It is a good idea, as well, to keep track of the number of calories you save each weekend over a period of a month. Keeping in mind that 3,500 calories make up a pound of fat, see how many pounds you have not added to your present weight just by substituting on the weekends. If you just stay the same, you'll be better off; but you won't stay the same. If you are serious about watching portion size, enjoying your selections, and keeping your health in mind, you will lose weight—and even enjoy losing it. We will return to this principle of food substitution when we talk about the Control Plan in the next chapter— once your weight has stabilized. At this point in time you don't want to use the substitution plan for every day, since you want to lose. Using it on weekends will still allow you to lose when you combine it with the Five-Day Plan during the week.

11

Staying Thin: A Weigh of Life

WELCOME: WHAT'RE YOUR CHANCES?

You'll be glad to know that the outlook for obese adolescents is not so bleak as you may have believed. Getting there and staying there are sides of the same coin—and it isn't necessary to keep flipping from one side to the other.

A recent five-to ten-year followup of forty-five patients who had participated in a weight-loss program during their adolescence revealed that more than half of them were no longer obese. These were all people who, as teenagers, had been treated at a time when they were all at least 20 percent over their desired weight. The followup was done when the patients were between eighteen and twenty-seven years old.

Treatment consisted of individualized nutrition counseling, behavior modification, exercise programs, and supportive counseling, and the patients were put on a diet of 1,000 to 1,400 calories per day.

Followup studies are interesting. Men lost less absolute weight than women did but had a greater reduction in percent over their desired weight because of their greater growth in height. I made this point earlier in an attempt to keep girls from getting discouraged—girls should not run the weight-loss race with boys.

The end result of this study showed that twenty-two patients had lost more than twenty pounds each and fifteen had lost twenty pounds or less. Twenty-eight patients were no longer obese and twelve patients were no longer overweight.

So chances are better than hopeful—they are downright good. It isn't a case of here today, gone tomorrow, back again the day after. The "yo-yo" syndrome—an excuse to put back the weight you lost—is shown to be what I have always felt it to be, a method to string yourself along to get fat again. That needn't happen; it almost can't happen if you follow the simple method for control that I have devised for you.

At the end of the book I've included some easy-to-prepare and tasty low-calorie recipes that will help you vary your diet and stave off boredom. You may even want to experiment in the kitchen and create your own low-calorie dishes. However, it is true that most people who are thin eat pretty much the same foods, prepared pretty much the same way every day, so you can easily stick to a more prosaic diet to lose or control your weight, and not bother with any of these menus. But if you find you want to spice up your meals, you may enjoy some of the low-calorie treats I've included.

MAINTAINING YOUR WEIGHT

The first thing to do is to take a good hard look at what you have done. Make out a chart on a piece of paper so you can evaluate your progress to date. It should look something like this:

Name:_____

Date:_____

When I began this weight-loss plan:_____

When I ended this weight-loss plan:_____

Number of total inches lost:
(in the areas I asked you to measure)_____

Number of total pounds lost:_____

Average number of pounds lost per week:_____

Following are some instructions to help you maintain weight loss.

1. Weigh yourself daily and record your weight. Previously, while you were on the diet, I wanted you to stay off the scale as much as possible, limiting your weighing to no more than once a week. Now, however, you must weigh every day, though *only once.* The best time to do it is on arising, nude, after urinating. This is basically your true weight. It will fluctuate from this figure throughout the day. Don't drive yourself (and everyone else in the house) crazy by constantly getting on the scale. If you forget to weigh yourself in the morning, forget it. Relax. Cool it. You'll be all right.

2. Should you see that you are putting on weight, get back on one of the diet plans immediately. Don't wait. If you wait you'll likely gain more.

3. Don't let social obligations get in the way of your weight.

4. Drink your eight eight-ounce glasses of water a day.

5. Develop for yourself some form of exercise program. You can join a group if you prefer. Many teens and adolescents go to weight camps over the summer specifically for this endeavor. It's a good idea. It is important, however, that you don't make your exercise program into a torture. Then all you will be thinking about are ways to get out of it.

6. Take your multivitamin capsule once a day without fail.

7. Remember the principle of eating only when you are hungry. Adhere to this to the very best of your ability.

8. Try not to eat large amounts of food shortly before bedtime. In fact, the less you eat before going to bed at night, the better. It is not true that you will thereby feel hungry in the morning.

9. Remember that, in general, food generates hunger. The more you eat, the more of an urge you are likely to have to continue to eat.

10. Eat slowly. Take small bites, chew well, put your knife and fork down while chewing.

11. Don't do anything when you eat except enjoy your food. Reading, watching TV, arguing, etc., are out. These activities will distract you from your primary concern at the time: attention to your food.

Finally, there is the matter of what to eat. By now you have at last gotten down to a weight you can live with. It may not be your ideal weight—that might have been an impossible dream to begin with—but it is far from the weight you once were. What you must keep in mind, now, is that you will always be watching your weight. For as long as you live. Because if you do not watch it, you will gain it back. You will be eating food that is tasty and enjoyable; you can eat junk food, even pretzels and peanuts, if you just follow the simple directions for the Control Calculator.

THE CONTROL CALCULATOR

This is a very simple device—a measurement to tell you about the specific relationship between you and what you eat. Hopefully you now understand the changed eating habits I have fostered in you over this period of time. You will now use this new behavioral modification with the Control Calculator to choose among a greater variety of foods without putting on any extra weight. Here's how it works:

The average, routinely active person utilizes between 10 and 15 calories per pound of body weight each day to satisfy energy requirements. If you live a more rugged life involving a good deal of sports or other physical exertion, you may have to add calories to this figure. You will know this by checking your daily weight.

Age is a factor in the Control Calculator. The older you get, the fewer calories your body demands. Unfortunately, habit patterns never age. They stay as youthful as ever. So you must always be on the alert for a possible relapse into them. Keep your pictures on hand to remind you of what these old habit patterns did to you once. They will do it to you again if you do not follow the principles of control.

Now, let us adjust your weight. Let us take your new weight of X pounds and multiply it by the average between 10 and 15 calories per pound that is the amount of energy the average person spends to stay at normal weight. That is a point where food intake and energy output equal out. This figure we will take as 12 calories per pound. Multiply 12 times X (your weight) and the figure you come up with is your caloric number.

THE CALORIC NUMBER

What exactly is your Caloric Number? Let us say you have lost approximately twenty pounds and are at your "normal" weight of 115. In order to determine what your caloric requirement is, you multiply your new weight of 115 by the average number 12 (between 10 and 15 calories per pound of body weight). The number you come up with is 1,380, which represents the number of calories you can take in each day and, hopefully, stay the weight you are now. You can take these calories from any type of food—peanuts, popcorn, ice cream, etc.—but remember these calories from carbohydrate foods add up pretty quickly and won't leave you room for much real food. I suggest that you spend your caloric number wisely, as though it were an allowance you had to spend on important articles. However you spend it, you should not exceed it, or you will start re-gaining weight. It is not a good idea to have to keep trying to lose one day for the excesses of the day before. Somehow you never catch up.

Using your Caloric Number wisely will bring you all sorts of dividends. You can eat the same items your friends may be eating (you just don't have to eat the same amount); you can eat the healthier types of food as well. And you can do all this without gaining weight.

Your Caloric Number may change as you get older; you may find that it takes less food to maintain it. This is not an unnatural occurrence. The Caloric Number is not a fixed identity, but it will give you a valuable point of reference in your relationship with food.

You should use the charts of food substitutes provided earlier in this book—when we discussed weekend eating—from which to select your meals. You may certainly add items to this listing, provided you make sure you know the proper calories involved. As long as you follow these instructions, you need never be fat again.

PEANUTS, POPCORN

These items tempt many kids who are trying to lose weight. Of the two, peanuts are the more dangerous. An ounce of these nuts, dry-roasted, will furnish about 175 calories. That may not sound like much, but can anyone stop after eating just an ounce of peanuts? If your child is a peanut addict, at least make it more difficult for him to get at them. If you are going to have them in the house at all, at least have them in the shell. You needn't cooperate with the food industry to make it as easy as possible to get to the food. The food industry wants to make eating, nibbling, munching, crunching almost a reflex activity. Open a can or a jar or a box—and there the food is. The act of shelling peanuts means involving one's hands, relating to what one is eating, slowing down the actual eating of the food by placing a barrier in the way. You would be surprised how many fewer nuts are consumed once one has to shell them. Talk about the old shell game . . . here's a new use for it.

Popcorn is another matter. This particular "junk" item comes in three basic fashions: plain (that is, without butter or salt), butter or cheese flavored, and caramel coated. This last is considered a candy and I would like to exclude it from this particular discussion. However, popcorn, at its most buttery, is usually no more than 50 calories per cup, and at its least buttery, about 30. In addition to providing so few calories it serves the exquisite purpose of filling you up. What is most dangerous about popcorn is the great amount of salt many people sprinkle over it. Since salt also makes one thirsty, you drink—usually either diet soda, Coke, or water. Any of these fluids at such a time is not helpful to your weight. Coke with its high sugar content will add fat to your already bulging collection; however, all these drinks add fluid and the salt keeps these fluids locked into the body, thereby putting on almost immediate weight.

So if you are going to eat popcorn as a "junk" interlude—and it's not such a bad idea, after all is said and done—the best way to indulge is to take it plain. One or two cupfuls every now and then to satisfy the "munchies" and you'll get filled up as well.

But if you must salt, use salt substitute, and heaven knows there are enough of these around, and use a minimum of margarine instead of butter. It isn't that margarine has fewer calories than butter—they run about the same ounce for ounce—but margarine has less fat content and it is this, as well as calories, that you want to avoid.

JUNK FOODS AND HEALTH FOODS

You can't always tell these items apart. Not all junk foods are junk; not all health foods are virtuous. A case in point is the cheeseburger, on which so many fast food corporations depend so greatly. A cheeseburger once in a while, or even twice a week, is not such a bad thing. It is mostly meat, cheese, onion, lettuce, tomato, and a bun. If you stay away from the deep-fried potatoes and the onion rings, you aren't doing so badly calorie-wise and you have the security of knowing that you aren't all that different from your peers. The problem in this is in overindulgence; that's really what makes most junk foods fit for junkies. The advertising helps. "Who can eat one potato chip or one pretzel?" asks Madison Avenue. Well, surprise, surprise—you can. Maybe not one but half a dozen, if you put your mind to it. And not every day but maybe once a week, just often enough to know that you aren't a freak, that you do have some measure of control over your environment. It isn't necessary, it isn't essential—and, if you are worried about losing "control," then you had best avoid the experiment—but I can assure you that this brainwashing the ad agencies have done concerning food is all wrong. And sooner or later you have to understand that the only person properly in charge of your head is you. Granted this is a fairly sophisticated approach, but adolescents and teens are more sophisticated these days. One's own evaluation of what one is doing wrong is worth more than anyone else's. That is what I have been trying to get you to do in these pages: evaluate your behavior and, hopefully, change it.

Just to give you an idea how publicity about food changes our lives, take a standard "health" food, spinach. I have nothing against spinach; it is a fine vegetable. But to try to make something magical about it, to stand it apart from other foods in this respect, is a misappropriation of options. Contrary to what Popeye has been telling kids about the powers of spinach, it's nearly worthless as a source of iron in the diet. What started all the good press was a typographic error in a turn-of-the-century nutrition book that showed the iron content in spinach as ten times higher than its true value. The error has been perpetuated in nutritional guides ever since. Actually, the iron that spinach contains is not readily usable by the body. Half-truths and wish-fulfillments are responsible for most ingredients in our diets today. Faced by such a mass of confusion and conflicting opinions, it is necessary to be thoughtful, weigh the evidence as presented, and pick and choose for yourself to obtain the desired goal of getting thin.

Careful planning of a diet, as I have shown, can include some of the "so-called" junk foods. These foods usually have increased quantities of fats as well as increased quantities of simple sugars and allowances must be made for them by canceling out other items in the diet. The problem is more one of the child at the doctor's office who looks at his diet and says, "Do I eat this stuff before or after my regular food?" "Regular foods," must now, in many cases, become occasional foods, and positive thinking take the place of poor nutritional habits. It's not hard to do.

It's much easier, in fact, than staying fat.

A FINAL WORD

When you are not hungry, don't eat. If there is one piece of advice I would like you to take away from these pages, it is that. Even if you have not approached your Caloric Number for any particular day, that doesn't mean you have to eat something just because "you've got it coming."

It all comes down to hunger, at last. If your hunger to be thin is greater than your momentary hunger for food, you need never worry about being fat again. Remember to always ask yourself the question: "Am I hungry?" And wait for the answer before you start to eat.

One of the favorite expressions of the day is "Give me a

break!'' I hope that in this book, I've given you one. You the overweight kid, and you the worried parent. If I have done my job at all well, I have shown both of you how to put a brake on the eating cycle that is probably consuming you fairly equally.

Want a break?

You've got one.

Appendix: Low-Calorie Recipes

BREAKFASTS

RIVIERA TOAST:
(1 serving, 110 calories)

No breakfast item but this when used.

1 egg
Salt substitute
¼ teaspoon ground
  cinnamon
½ teaspoon liquid sugar
  substitute
⅛ cup unsweetened
  pineapple juice
1½ slices whole-wheat bread
2 tablespoons diet
  margarine

Beat the eggs until light, then add salt substitute to taste; the cinnamon, sugar substitute, and pineapple juice ingredients and beat thoroughly. Soak the bread well in this mixture, then sauté in the margarine heated in a heavy skillet until brown on both sides. Serve hot.

NOTE: This can sometimes go as a brunch on weekends and serve for lunch and breakfast. If so, you can add a slice of pineapple to each slice of bread.

THE BIG APPLE PANCAKE
(1 serving, 195 calories)

1 apple
1 egg

Peel the apple, then core it and slice into thin strips. Bring the ap-

¼ *cup bread crumbs (any)*
1 *teaspoon fresh lemon juice*
¼ *teaspoon ground
cinnamon*
½ *liquid sugar substitute*
½ *cup skim milk*

ple slices to a simmer with the lemon juice, sweetener, and spice. Test the apple with a fork to make sure it is tender.

Combine the egg, bread crumbs, and skim milk in a blender; blend. Combine the blended mixture with the cooked apple. In a nonstick pan, over medium heat, ladle in the batter to make pancakes. Brown first one side, then the other.

NOTE: You may serve a small amount of any low-calorie jam to add to the taste of this breakfast. With the above dish you may have nothing else for the meal.

You Can Risk It for this Biscuit
(3 servings, 90 calories each)

Yes, you can even have a breakfast biscuit occasionally if you follow this recipe. Here's what it takes:

2 *tablespoons diet
margarine*
½ *cup unsweetened orange
juice*
¼ *cup liquid sugar
substitute*
1 *teaspoon grated orange
rind*
Commercial biscuit dough
½ *teaspoon ground
cinnamon*

Combine the margarine, orange juice, sweetener, and grated rind in a saucepan and heat just until the margarine melts and the mixture is well blended. Pour into a baking pan and roll out the biscuit dough fairly thin. Sprinkle the cinnamon over the dough, then roll up. Cut the dough into equal slices. Place the slices, close together, in the orange syrup. Bake in a preheated hot oven (450° F) for 20 to 25 minutes, until golden brown. Have with skim milk.

Popeyed Spinach Omelet
(1 serving, 90 calories)

If you don't like spinach, this works equally well with asparagus.

2 tablespoons well-drained chopped cooked spinach
1 egg, beaten with 1 teaspoon water
Salt substitute or seasoned pepper to taste
2 tablespoons all-purpose flour

Mix everything together very well. Make sure your nonstick omelet pan is nice and hot, then pour the egg mixture carefully in. Cook, lifting the edge of the cooked egg to let the uncooked egg run underneath. Turn out onto a heated plate, folding the omelet over as you turn. Serve at once.

This will take care of breakfast completely.

Oatmeal That's a Meal
(4 servings, 100 calories each)

This one, also, makes you a complete breakfast. You'll really feel your oats with this recipe.

2 tablespoons diet margarine
1 cup skim milk
¾ cup rolled instant oats
½ cup grated cheese
Dash of dry mustard
2 tablespoons chopped pimiento
½ teaspoon salt substitute
2 slices well-done beef bacon, crumbled
2 eggs, separated

Add the margarine to the milk in a saucepan and heat to simmering over direct heat. Now add the oats and cook for 5 minutes, stirring constantly. Remove from the heat and stir in the cheese. When the cheese melts, add the mustard, pimiento, salt substitute, bacon, and the egg yolks, beaten. Beat the whites until they are stiff and then fold the oat mixture into the whites. Turn into a greased casserole and bake in a preheated moderately slow oven (about 325° F) for nearly 1 hour.

LUNCHES

Here are some creative selections for a little later in the day. These can all but furnish a complete lunch.

SALMON SURPRISE
(3 servings, 120 calories each)

1 can (1 pound) pink or red salmon
1 tablespoon fresh lemon juice
Dash of cayenne
1 teaspoon salt substitute
2 eggs, beaten
⅔ cup chopped celery
1 cup bread crumbs
½ teaspoon all-purpose flour
½ cup skim milk
½ cup water

Drain the salmon; discard the skin and bones but save ½ cup of the juice. Flake the fish, then add the remaining ingredients, including the salmon liquid, and mix well. Pack the mixture firmly into a greased glass loaf pan. Bake in a moderate over (350° F) until brown and firm, from 30 to 40 minutes.

NOTE: This is good served plain or with canned tomato soup, undiluted, as a suace. You shouldn't need anything else for lunch.

TEENAGE CHEESEBURGER
(3 servings, 260 calories each)

This is a burger emperor, let alone king. One of these should do nicely for lunch.

¾ pound ground beef
2 tablespoons skim milk or water
⅓ teaspoon salt substitute

Mix the ground beef with the milk, salt substitute, and pepper. Form into 6 patties about 3 inches in diameter. Cut cheese into 6 pieces

Dash of pepper
3 slices American cheese
¼ cup chili sauce
1½ tablespoons pickle relish
1 teaspoon prepared
    mustard or prepared
    horseradish
2 tablespoons diet
    margarine or oil (except if
    using a nonstick pan)
Thin slices whole-wheat
    bread

slightly smaller than the meat patties. Mix the chili sauce, pickle relish, and mustard or horseradish thoroughly. Melt the margarine in a skillet and pan-fry the patties slowly 10 to 15 minutes, turning them several times as they cook. Place on the toasted bread (one slice is all you require for each burger), spread with the piquant sauce, and top with a slice of cheese. Broil until the cheese begins to melt. Serve with things you know you can eat: green onions, radishes, celery, etc. I like it with lettuce and a slice of tomato as well.

GETTING AHEAD SALAD (3 servings, 135 calories each)

You can start this lunch with a glass of tomato juice and conclude it with a glass of skim milk. We'll be using a head of cauliflower or broccoli for the main course.

1 small head cauliflower or
    broccoli
½ cup vinegar and oil
    dressing
½ cup grated sharp cheese
Crisp lettuce or endive

Separate the cauliflower into flowerets and soak about 1 hour in cold water to which 1 teaspoon salt substitute has been added. Drain and cook, uncovered, in rapidly boiling water (with salt substitute added) 6 to 8 minutes, or until barely tender. Drain, cool and pour the vinegar and oil dressing over the vegetable. Let it stand 30 minutes in the refrigerator, then add the cheese and toss together thoroughly. Serve chilled, on crisp lettuce leaves.

Don't Skimp on Shrimp Cocktail
(3 to 4 servings, 150 calories each)

This one is an old standby for many of us former fatties; I still enjoy it with the slightly different twist I've given it here. You can start your lunch with a bowl of Campbell's clam chowder and finish with a can of any diet soda.

1 pound shrimp, cleaned and cooked
½ cup chili sauce
½ teaspoon prepared horseradish
¼ teaspoon Worcestershire sauce
¼ teaspoon fresh lemon juice
⅓ cup diced celery
⅓ cup diced green pepper
Crisp lettuce

Chill the cooked and cleaned shrimp thoroughly. Combine all the other ingredients except the lettuce and mix with the shrimp. Serve in small sherbet glasses or cups lined with the lettuce leaves. Eat slowly. Shrimp are nice chewy items, so make the most of them.

Settling Your Hash
(2 servings, 280 calories each)

Hash is another long-time favorite "diet" food. Again, it need not be a bland and characterless "fill in," as I'm sure you'll agree if you give this one a try.

1 cup beef broth or 1 bouillon cube in 1 cup boiling water
2 cups grated raw cauliflower
1 medium onion, grated
½ pound diced cooked beef
1 teaspoon salt substitute
2 tablespoons corn oil

Combine the broth, cauliflower, onion, beef, and salt substitute and put into a heavy skillet along with the oil. Cover and simmer 25 to 30 minutes, or until the cauliflower and onion are well cooked and the hash is slightly browned on the underside. Add more water if the hash becomes dry. Uncover the skillet and place in a moderate oven (350° F) 15 to 20 minutes longer. Remove from the oven and fold the hash over omelet fashion. Place on a hot platter, using a wide spatula or turner.

NOTE: A glass of diet soda or skim milk should complete the meal.

DINNER

There are plenty of choices here if you just use a little imagination. Here are a few of them:

A ROLL OF STEAK
(4 servings, 355 calories each)

1½ pounds round steak, cut ½ inch thick
¼ chopped onion
¼ cup corn oil
1 cup bread crumbs
½ teaspoon sage
¼ cup fresh celery, finely chopped
1 bouillon cube dissolved in 1¼ cups boiling water
1 egg, beaten
Salt substitute and pepper to taste

Wipe the meat thoroughly with a damp cloth and pound it all over vigorously with the edge of a heavy saucer. Sauté the onion in the oil until it turns yellow; add to the bread crumbs and combine lightly with all the remaining ingredients. If the crumbs are excessively dry (this is a matter of taste), more liquid may be added. Spread this dressing over the steak and roll the meat up like a jelly roll. Secure it by tying it at the ends and the center with string. Brown on all sides in a small amount of fat in a skillet; add ½ cup hot water, cover tightly and bake in a moderately slow oven (about 325° F), 1 hour, or until the meat is very tender. Remove the meat roll to a hot platter. Remove the string and keep the meat hot while making gravy from the skillet drippings for the members of the family who are not overweight. For the fat kid, the steak and a couple of vegetables with a small salad will be plenty.

A Deal of Veal
(6 servings, 275 calories each)

2½ pounds veal
3 tablespoons diet
   margarine
1 medium onion, chopped
⅓ cup chopped celery
1½ teaspoons salt substitute

Wipe the veal with a damp cloth. Brown on one side in the margarine in a heavy kettle or Dutch oven. Turn the meat over and add the onion and celery, stirring the vegetables occasionally until the meat is well browned. Sprinkle the meat with salt substitute. Add about ½ cup hot water, cover tightly and simmer until meat is tender, about 1½ hours. Serve with a small tossed salad, a cup of boiled white rice, and what better deal can you get?

In Tune with Tuna
(3 servings, 372 calories each)

1½ cups skim milk
1 tablespoon diet margarine
1 cup bread crumbs
1 tablespoon grated onion
½ teaspoon salt substitute

Heat the milk very hot in a saucepan, then add the margarine, crumbs, salt substitute, celery, and the tuna. The egg yolks should be well beaten and a little of the hot

1 cup diced celery
1 large can water-packed
   tuna, drained and flaked
3 eggs, separated
1 tablespoon lemon juice

mixture stirred in; then return it to the saucepan and heat it for about 3 minutes or until it is thickened, stirring constantly so it doesn't burn. Remove it from the heat and fold in the lemon juice and stiffly beaten egg whites. Turn into a lightly margarine-greased casserole and bake in a preheated moderately slow oven (325° F)1 hour, or until a knife inserted in the center comes out clean.

NOTE: If desired, the celery may be cooked in a small amount of boiling water for 5 minutes before combining with the other ingredients; otherwise it will remain slightly crisp even after baking.

MEAL ON A SKEWER
(2 to 3 servings, 450 calories each)

The preparation here is a bit lengthy but it's worth it. You can also take out some of your frustrations during the time.

1 pound lamb (or other
   meat), cut into chunks a
   little larger than bite size
Marinade: Lemon juice,
   Worcestershire sauce,
   ketchup, bay leaf,
   Campbell's tomato soup
   (undiluted), salt
   substitute, pepper (I use
   the tomato soup as a base
   and mix in the other
   ingredients to taste)

Marinate the meat in a closed dish for several hours (you can start it the day before). Stir the marinate occasionally to make certain all the meat is marinated evenly. String the ingredients in alternate fashion on skewers: meat, onion, pepper, mushroom, tomato. If you wish you can parboil the pepper and onion first; if not, stringing them as they are will provide a less cooked vegetable but one that is equally

Tomato
Raw onion
Green pepper
Mushrooms

tasty. When the skewers are all prepared, place them in pans in the oven at 325° F and roast, turning the skewers occasionally to make sure all sides of the meat get done equally. Serve hot. A complete dinner.

GOURMET HAMBURGERS
(4 servings, 250 calories each)

1 pound ground lean beef
(sirloin or round)
½ teaspoon salt
⅓ cup canned sliced
mushrooms, drained
¼ cup dry sherry

Blend the beef and the salt. Form into 4 patties. Heat the pan and sprinkle it generously with pepper. Brown the beef on both sides; add the mushrooms and sherry. Simmer about 5 minutes, or to preferred doneness.

SAVORY CHICKEN LIVERS
(2 servings, 225 calories each)

1 package (8 ounces) frozen
chicken livers, defrosted
Dash of onion salt
1 teaspoon all-purpose flour
2 tomatoes, coarsely diced
1 teaspoon butter

Season the livers with the onion salt and sprinkle with the flour. Arrange alternating layers of tomatoes and livers in a shallow pan. Dot with butter and bake in a preheated 350° F oven about 20 minutes, or until the livers are done.

BROILED CHICKEN PAPRIKA
(4 servings, 200 calories each)

1 broiler (1½ to 2 pounds),
quartered

Sprinkle the chicken pieces generously with seasonings. Place 5

Onion salt
Paprika
Garlic powder

inches from the heat in a preheated broiler, skin side up. Broil 15 minutes. Turn and broil another 20 minutes, or until the chicken is done.

LOW CALORIE SALAD DRESSING
(1 cup, 12 calories per 2-tablespoon serving)

⅓ cup water
2 tablespoons all-purpose flour
½ cup vinegar
1 teaspoon liquid sugar substitute
½ teaspoon paprika
1 teaspoon prepared horseradish
1 teaspoon dry mustard
½ teaspoon Worcestershire sauce
¼ cup ketchup
Dash of garlic powder

Blend the water, flour, and vinegar in a saucepan. Cook and stir over low heat until smooth and thickened. Cool. Add the remaining ingredients; beat until smooth. Store, covered, in the refrigerator. Stir well before using.

AMBROSIA
(1 serving, 130 calories)

1 medium orange, peeled and sliced
¼ cup unsweetened orange juice
1 tablespoon shredded coconut

Arrange the orange slices in a serving dish, pour the orange juice over them and sprinkle with coconut. Chill.

CRUNCHY DIP FOR TV
SNACK OR COCKTAIL DIP
(½ cup, 12 calories per
tablespoon)

¼ cup cottage cheese
¼ cup finely chopped
cucumber
1 teaspoon finely chopped
onion or chives
½ cup grated raw carrot
1 tablespoon chili sauce
Dash each of salt, pepper,
and celery salt

Blend together all the ingredients. Store in the refrigerator; it will keep for several days.

ORANGE DESSERT
(6 servings, 12 calories
each)

1 envelope unflavored
gelatin
1¾ cups cold water
1 tablespoon grated orange
rind
¼ cup unsweetened orange
juice
Sweetening substitute
equivalent to 4 teaspoons
sugar
2 egg whites

Sprinkle the gelatin over ¼ cup of the water in a small cup. Bring the remaining 1½ cups of water to a boil in a small saucepan; add the orange rind and simmer 2 minutes. Add the softened gelatin and stir until the gelatin is dissolved. Stir in the orange juice and sweetening. Strain; chill until the mixture mounds slightly when dropped from a spoon. Beat the egg whites stiff and fold them into the gelatin mixture. Turn into a 1-quart mold or 6 individual molds. Chill until firm.

Index